Heart and Soul

HOW TO SHAPE UP THE BODY AND THE SPIRIT

KAREN THOMPSON,
MHA, BSN, RN-CV

Publishing Designs, Inc.
P. O. Box 3241
Huntsville, Alabama 35810

Editors: Debra G. Wright, Peggy Coulter

Cover and Interior Design: CrosslinCreative.net
Cover image: LightStock
Interior images: Creative Market, BigStock

Printed in the United States of America

Publisher's Cataloging-in-Publication Data

Thompson, Karen, 1960—

Heart and Soul / Karen Thompson

158 pp.

13 chapters and study questions

1. Physical and Spiritual Parallels. 2. Health Issues. 3. Christian—daily life

I. Title.

ISBN 978-1-945127-07-6

231

To my sweet grandchildren Skyler, Haley, Alana, and Aiden. Mimi loves you. May you make healthy choices and serve our Lord and Master always.

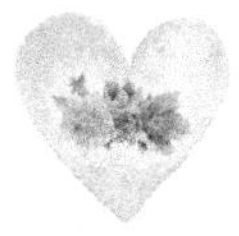

"Be not wise in your own eyes;
Fear the Lord and depart evil.
It will be health to your flesh,
And strength to your bones."
—Proverbs 3:7–8

Contents

Acknowledgments

Thank you, Mom, for making me promise I would write this book and being there in good times and bad. Thank you, Dad, for always challenging me to do better. Thank you to the Toledo Road and Cary Church of Christ congregations for your support. In addition, the ministers and elders at both places have been very encouraging and supporting. And thank you Cindy Colley for encouraging me to "Just write it!"

But most of all I must thank my dear husband Terry for his years of service and self-sacrifice to our Lord, serving as a humble elder, demonstrating unwavering love and support to me, during good times and bad. He is still my spiritual compass. Without him, I would be lost here and hereafter.

Finally, I'm grateful to my sweet family Chad, Jennifer, Danielle and Misha. May you also make healthy choices and remember to put Christ first in your life for all your decisions, no matter how big or small, and you will surely be blessed by Him.

Editors' Foreword

If you are getting ready to study this book, I'll tell you why you do not want to skip the introduction.

I first met Karen Hall Thompson in the early 1970s when I was 22 and had just started attending the Toledo Road Church of Christ in Lorain, Ohio. Karen was still in high school, so she was not really on my radar. However, I did get to know her parents, Billy Joe and Wanda Hall, who were part of a group of young married couples epitomizing the words "friendship evangelism." Because of their efforts and others, I became a Christian in 1976.

Karen's parents loved to sing and so did I. A favorite memory is of a group that gathered in the auditorium toward the end of potluck dinners, singing hymns. How those voices blended! Not only were Karen and her parents there, but one of those singers (and a frequent song leader) was Terry Thompson, Karen's future husband.

Soon I decided to attend a Christian college. After graduation, I began work in Nashville and lost track of Terry and Karen. So you can imagine my surprise when one of my first projects at Publishing Designs was to edit a book written by Karen Hall Thompson from North Carolina. Could this be the Karen Hall I knew in Lorain? I soon discovered that she was indeed!

Now, why shouldn't you skip the introduction? Because it unveils Karen and her journey toward *Heart and Soul.* She opens her own heart and shares some of the personal heartbreaks and triumphs she experienced regarding her own physical and spiritual health.

Heart and Soul will mean so much more to you if you take the time to read the introduction.

Editors sometimes get bogged down in all the minutia of grammar and style. I am guilty. But it was impossible to miss the star that came shining through in Karen's writings: *God needs healthy workers to do His work.*

May we all take to heart Karen's lessons on improving ourselves physically and spiritually.

Debra G. Wright, co-editor

So often we grab a book that looks appealing and then discover that we cannot relate to the lessons. Why? Could it be that we feel the author is preaching rather than sharing? A sales mentor once instructed, "We don't sell, we show and tell."

You are holding paper with words about the body and soul. But it's much more. You are holding the expertise of a health professional and an elder's wife who is sharing her story. Publishing Designs gladly presents *Heart and Soul* to you, in hopes that your heart and soul will be strengthened, and that you will show and tell others.

Peggy Coulter, co-editor

Introduction

Food for Thought

It is important to be proactive rather than reactive when it comes to your health. My goal in writing this book is twofold. I want to help sisters and their families whom I love so dearly to take control of their lives and improve themselves both physically and spiritually through prevention. Your mother was right. An ounce of prevention is worth a pound of cure.

Do you know that statistically the United States spends more per person for health care than any other country in the world?[1] Because of that wouldn't you expect our nation to be the healthiest? The World Health Organization measures health by lifespan, birth weight, and infant death rate statistics. In those matters, the United States is not ranked the best. Based on life expectancy it ranks thirty-fourth out of 191 countries.[2]

It may surprise you to find out the number one health threat to our country is of our own doing—our lifestyle choices. We are bombarded with worldly marketing strategies that lead us to believe "life is good; live it up." But facts reveal that high blood pressure, high cholesterol, smoking, diabetes, poor diet, lack of physical activity, and obesity are the leading risk factors of the American lifestyle.[3]

Lack of exercise can lead to obesity.[4] Obesity can lead to high blood pressure and diabetes. Uncontrolled high blood pressure and diabetes can lead to chronic expensive diseases such as heart disease, stroke, and kidney failure requiring dialysis. High stress, on the job and in the home, acts as a catalyst and aggravates all of the above.[5]

Breast cancer and ovarian cancer may make the headlines these days but heart disease is still the number one cause of death in women.

There is so much misinformation out there that the First Friday in February has been designated "National Wear Red Day" by the American Heart Association and the National Heart, Lung and Blood Institute since 2003. Maybe you have noticed the "little red dress lapel pin"? That pin is meant to raise awareness to the fact that heart disease is not just a man's disease.

Heart disease is the number one cause of death in women in the United States.[6] And I am convinced that "heart disease" is the biggest threat to the church as well. Our selfish pursuits, egged on by society, often bog us down so much that we become inactive in the church. Our fascination and pursuit of material things—entertainment, dining out, improving our appearance—consume our time and paychecks and lead us away from our God-given roles in service as grandmothers, mothers, wives, daughters, and sisters.

If you do not believe me, open your checkbook and follow the money trail. You may be surprised where your paycheck is really going. Compare this to what you are giving to God and to others. Your heart tells on you. "As in water face reflects face, so a man's heart reveals the man" (Proverbs 27:19).

Spiritual Starvation

We are spiritually malnourished and starved as well. Worse, we are starving our families. We look for worldly rather than godly ways to solve our problems and ease our pain, especially in the form of alcohol, prescription drugs, and illegal substances. This road leads to spiritual disability and death.

The great news is we have control over all these risk factors for heart disease both physically and spiritually. God will help us. "But without faith it is impossible to please Him, for he who comes to God must believe that He is, and that He is a rewarder of those who diligently seek Him" (Hebrews 11:6). What will we choose?

1. A physical life limited and shortened by fatigue, shortness of breath, and pain from being obese and inactive?
2. A spiritually overweight life burdened down with worldly concerns about our appearance, home decor, and the stress of keeping up with the Joneses?
3. A life of peace?

Surprise!

My family threw me a surprise birthday party in 2010. It was great being with family and friends. But after looking at the pictures taken that day, I had to face the fact that I was fat. I was a health-care provider and knew better. How did this happen?

The weight gain sneaked up on me over an eight- to 10-year period, and I tried to deny it.

- Five pounds for Christmas and Thanksgiving.
- Five to 10 pounds during the time my grandmother suffered and
- died from cancer.
- Five to 10 pounds with the grief and loss of good friends because of relocations.
- Five to 10 pounds during a series of personal disappointments on the job and with close family and friends.

I allowed grief, loss, disappointment, and relationship difficulties to drive me to try to fill the hole in my heart with food. I then became more socially isolated and inactive, allowing work-related activities to consume my time. Next thing I knew I was up 70 pounds and had developed high blood pressure and high blood sugar readings in the 300s—three times the normal.

I am happy to report that with some serious self-evaluation and physical and spiritual goal setting, I was able to lose 70 pounds and come off blood pressure and diabetic medication. This required prayer, exercise, strict calorie counting, food monitoring, and medical supervision for more than a year. My husband and I went on this journey together. I highly recommend the "buddy approach."

Heart and Soul Fit for Service

When traveling to Costa Rica, the Spanish words, *pura vida,* greeted us everywhere. In the simplest form these words mean "pure life" in English. The "Ticos," Costa Ricans, have adopted the idea that a pure and simple life can be peaceful and joyful in this motto, *pura vida.* True peace and joy can only be found in service to our Lord.

Healthy Hearts

In an average cardiac rehab program, a heart patient will spend about 12 weeks exercising and attending classes to learn to recognize and manage risk factors and then set attainable goals before discharge. My prayer for you is that over the next few weeks, you will learn to recognize and manage your own risk factors and set attainable goals by spending time studying God's words, not mine. You will learn to exercise your physical and your spiritual heart to get healthy.

A lean muscular heart, body, and soul will be strong and full of energy for the Lord. I personally know the consequences of sin. Too many times I have tried to stand on my own two feet, but now I realize that I am the strongest when I am on my knees. A close friend once quoted this passage to me: "Therefore humble yourselves under the mighty hand of God, that He might exalt you in due time, casting all your cares upon Him, for He cares for you" (1 Peter 5:6–7).

It is always good to teach what you know. I know about the burden of obesity and the trap of worldly pursuits. Hopefully we will get stronger together.

As a wellness nurse and program director of a local cardiac rehab program, I work with patients who deal with a multitude of heart-related problems and surgeries: stable angina, heart attacks, stents, bypass surgeries, valve replacements, heart failures, and heart transplants. My job is to help them adopt heart-healthy habits.

The importance of taking early preventive steps to control risk factors that might damage the heart has become clear to me. However, heart-healthy habits are even more critical for our spiritual heart health.

A plethora of information regarding your physical health and heart is available. Be careful of your sources. Remember, "The wisdom of this world is foolishness with God" (1 Corinthians 3:19).

However, we are going to spend time looking at what God's Word says about the spiritual heart, your mind, and your body. Paul says, "Set your mind on things above, not on things on the earth" (Colossians 3:2). The Lord told Jeremiah, "I, the Lord, search the heart, I test the mind, even to give every man according to his ways, according to the fruit of his doings" (Jeremiah 17:10). I wonder, does God search the heart and test the mind of a man today or did that occur only during the Old Testament times?

In the following chapters, we will review risk factors for physical and spiritual heart disease. Begin today to stretch your spiritual muscles by studying Solomon's step-by-step guide for soul improvement found in Proverbs 3.

Solomon had been blessed by God for his humble attitude and request for wisdom rather than riches. He was rewarded with both riches and wisdom more than anyone who has ever or will ever live. In Proverbs 3 Solomon taught his children to trust in God's wisdom and commandments rather than their own. He told them if they obeyed, not only would they be blessed with peace, long life, and prosperity but also health to their flesh and bones. Only they could make that choice.

The choices you make in life about what you eat, what you do, how you spend your time and money, and who your friends are, have physical and ultimately eternal, spiritual consequences. Those choices affect your heart and soul. From the perspective of a cardiac rehab and wellness specialist, my goal is to help you identify your risk factors and set realistic goals to successfully overcome risks. Ultimately, we will study what the Great Physician, our Lord Jesus Christ, has prescribed, and we will learn to take our medicine.

Karen Thompson
January 8, 2018

1

Realize That Less Is More

"Daniel purposed in his heart that he would not defile himself with the portion of the king's delicacies, nor with the wine which he drank" (Daniel 1:8).

Supersized Meals

Too many indulgences in carbs and sweets can lead to obesity. Obesity kills people of both genders and all ages and races. That includes workers in the Lord's church. As mentioned in the introduction, our own lifestyle is our biggest health threat—in particular, our nutrition and our activity level.[7] Both are believed to be related to poor nutrition from junk foods, convenience processed foods, and supersized meals loaded with high saturated fats, salt, and sugar, all of which can lead to obesity. We are accustomed to rushing to our cars after work, picking up the kids, and driving to a fast-food restaurant for dinner. How bad can it be when it tastes so good? Right? Why not supersize it for a dollar? If there are leftovers, we can just heat those up tomorrow. Unfortunately, this pattern becomes a habit and then a lifestyle.

Obesity is on the rise in my state. Obesity is on the rise in our entire nation as well, costing millions of dollars in health-care costs. Obesity is generally defined as a simple waist circumference measurement over the hips and around the belly button of greater than 35 inches in a non-pregnant woman.

There are two other ways to determine if your weight and body fat are a problem.

1. A simple BMI (Body Mass Index) is your weight (in kilograms) divided by your height (in meters) squared. When used as a screening tool, it will provide you with a "jumping off place" to identify a recommended weight range. To use the free National Institute of Health BMI graph or application, all you need is your height in inches and weight in pounds. For adults, a BMI of 18.5–24.9 is considered healthy. A BMI of 30 or higher is considered obese. Please note if you are extremely muscular, BMI may not be a good indicator of fat or health risks.
2. A skilled person painlessly "pinches" the skin with calipers. Fat percentages and lean muscle percentages can then be calculated and compared to age recommended determinations.

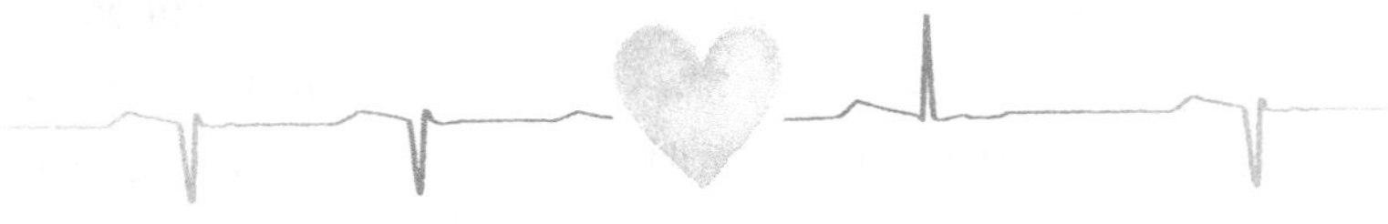

"You grew fat, you grew thick, you are obese! Then he forsook God who made him, and scornfully esteemed the Rock of his salvation" (Deuteronomy 32:15).

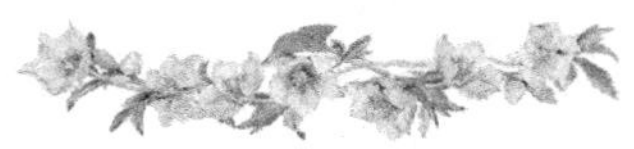

Burdened Hearts

Complications of obesity include high blood pressure and type 2 diabetes and can lead to stroke, coronary artery disease, and poor quality of life. Weight-related limitation in movement is a serious issue that can result in low self-esteem, depression, immobility, and potential dependence on others for self-care. Although this is not a lesson on weight loss, the Lord's church needs strong healthy women.

Heart disease is the number one killer of women in the United States right there along with men. We just develop it 10 years after men do.[8] Extra weight is a burden to both our physical and spiritual hearts, because it can slow us down. Weight management is a lifelong battle, so if you find yourself over the weight limit, nip it in the bud.

As previously mentioned, being overweight can raise your blood pressure. Normal textbook and American Heart Association guidelines recommend keeping blood pressure at 120/80 millimeters of mercury or lower. You will get a diagnosis of "hypertension," meaning too much pressure exerted on your inner artery walls, if your blood pressure is 140/90 or higher.[9] The top number, or systolic number, represents the pressure inside the arteries when the heart squeezes, and the bottom number represents the pressure inside the arteries when the heart is at rest (between beats).

Sometimes people under a doctor's care can come off their medicines, at least some of them, just by controlling their weight. As a practitioner in cardiac rehab, I have seen this over and over. As little as 5–10 percent of total body weight loss can make the difference. For example, if a 200-pound man loses 20 pounds,[10] it can make the difference in whether he needs his blood pressure medicines or diabetes medicines. This is great news and a wonderful benefit of weight loss. I have personally experienced this. About five years ago, I was obese and on the road to diabetes, high blood pressure, and ultimately heart disease.

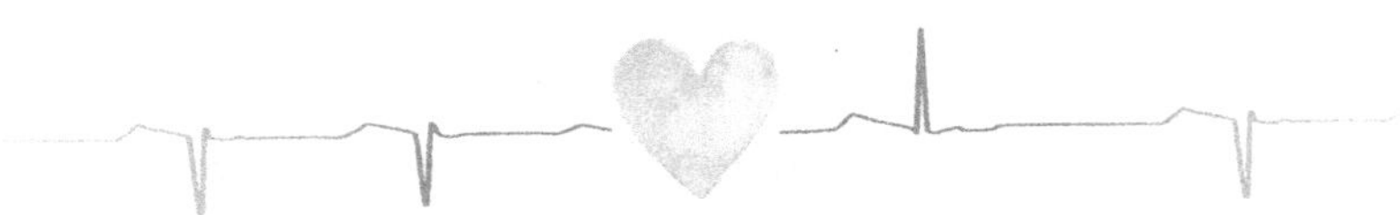

"The heart is deceitful above all things, and desperately wicked; who can know it? I, the Lord, search the heart, I test the mind, even to give every man according to his ways, according to the fruit of his doings" (Jeremiah 17:9–10).

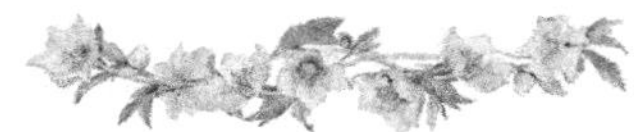

Preventive Eating

The DASH Diet (Dietary Approach to Stopping Hypertension) is a good way to reduce blood pressure.[11] Basically, this type of eating encourages fresh fruits and vegetables, rich in important electrolytes such as potassium, calcium, and magnesium. The diet promotes

- More fruits and vegetables
- Whole grain breads
- Lean meats (less processed)
- More fish and nuts
- Low-fat dairy
- Lower salt, meaning 1,500–2,400 milligrams per day (By the way, one level teaspoon of salt is about 1,500 milligrams.)
- Less saturated fats (fats that are solid at room temperature)

Many other diet plans incorporate these same basic heart healthy guidelines.

Daniel Refused Delicacies

Even in captivity, Daniel, "purposed in his heart" not to eat from the king's table. He chose instead to eat vegetables and drink water, long before the DASH Diet. King Nebuchadnezzar destroyed the temple at Jerusalem in 586 BC. A few years earlier, he captured some of the city's most intelligent young men and took them to Babylon to be trained in the language and literature of the Chaldeans. Four of these young men were Daniel, Shadrach, Meshach, and Abed-Nego. The king instructed his servant Ashpenaz to provide all these young men with the king's delicacies, the wine that he drank, and likely the meat that was sacrificed to idols.

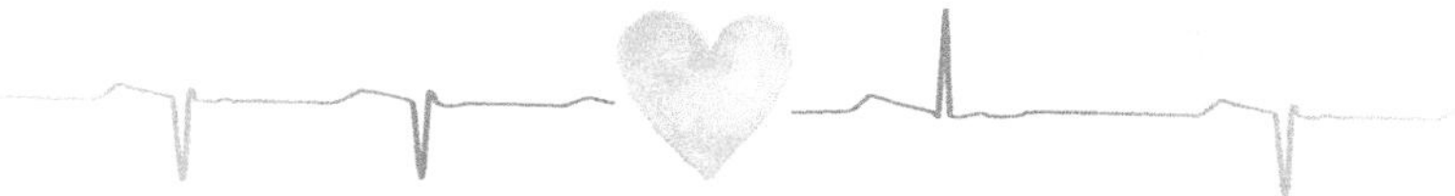

"Or do you not know that your body is the temple of the Holy Spirit who is in you, whom you have from God, and you are not your own? For you were bought at a price; therefore glorify God in your body and in your spirit, which are God's" (1 Corinthians 6:19–20).

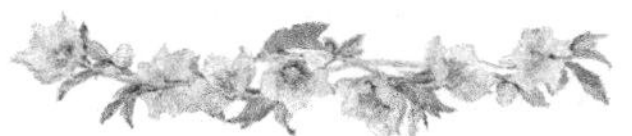

Daniel and his friends refused to drink the king's wine and eat of his delicacies, requesting to be fed vegetables and water instead. Ashpenaz fearfully but reluctantly agreed. After 10 days Daniel's group demonstrated better appearance, thinking, and health. They were found to be 10 times better. They stood up for their beliefs, and with God's help, they excelled in everything. Even under the stress of captivity, Daniel and his friends had a positive influence on their own nation as well as the Chaldeans during their captivity (Daniel 1:3–21).

Jesus said, "And do not fear those who kill the body but cannot kill the soul. But rather fear Him who is able to destroy both soul and body in hell" (Matthew 10:28). It took a lot of guts for Daniel, Shadrach, Meshach, and Abed-Nego to stand up to King Nebuchadnezzar. God rewarded them for their courage.

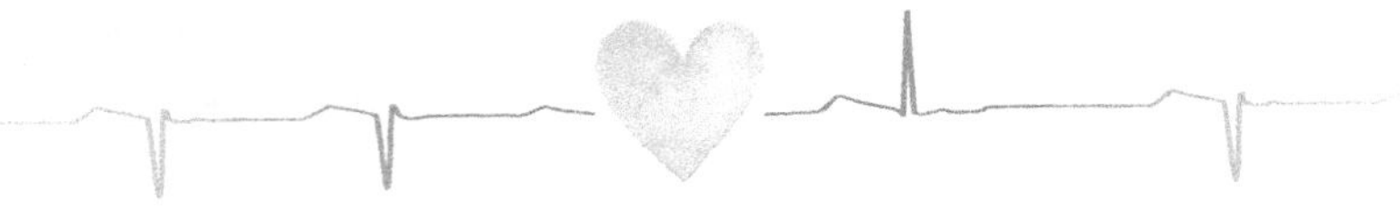

"And at the end of ten days their features appeared better and fatter in flesh than all the young men who ate the portion of the king's delicacies. Thus the steward took away their portion of delicacies and the wine that they were to drink, and gave them vegetables" (Daniel 1:15–16).

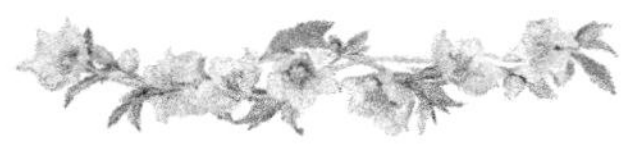

"Hyper" Tension

Hypertension or high blood pressure is considered a silent killer because it damages the inside of the arterial walls, making people more susceptible to clogging, clots, and cardiovascular disease.[12] If I took a high-pressure water hose and sprayed it onto a painted surface, what would happen to that painted surface after a short while? It would become pitted and marked. Similarly, the arterial walls of one with high blood pressure become vulnerable to clogging.

Most of the time people are not aware that their blood pressure is elevated, because they do not feel any symptoms. Medication might be necessary to bring down their blood pressure. Unfortunately, many people stop taking their medication because they do not feel any good effects from it. When I discover that a five-dollar medication could

Shaping up the Heart and Soul

By Karen Thompson MHA, BSN, RN-CV

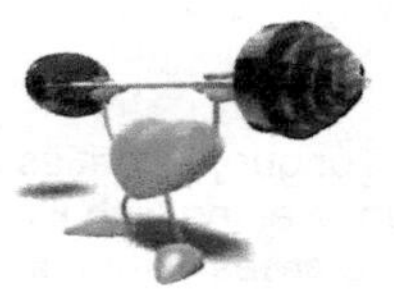

1. **Get Up and Go!**
   A. Christianity is **Active!** Jesus says- **Go** and **make** disciples of men Mat 28:19-20, **Walk** in the light Jn 12:35, **Stand United** Mar 3:24,
   B. Christianity requires **Discipline!** Paul says-Be **Diligent**, **Be** a good worker 2 Ti 2:15-19, **Run** the race, **throw** off the weights and **Keep** our eye on Jesus the author and finisher of our race. Heb12:1-2, **Run, Fight and be disciplined** to win the race. 1Co 9:24-27

2. **Choices**
   A. Mother is right! An **ounce** of Prevention is worth a **pound** of cure!
   B. Our choices Matter about what we put into our Mouths, Minds and Hearts
   C. Glorify God in your body and your spirit, which are God's 1 Co 6-19-20

3. **Exercise the Senses?**
   A. Your Words were found, and I ate them. Jer 15:16
   B. The Lord searches our hearts tests the mind Jer 17:10
   C. Taste and see that the Lord is good. Blessed is the man who trusts Him! Psa 34:8
   D. Lord's Promises. The righteous soul will not famish Pro 10:3 Those who trust in the Lord will have health to their flesh and strength to their bones Pro 3:5-8

4. **Preventing a Diseased and Burdened Heart**

A. Managing our Risk Factors like Stress, Nutrition, Body Weight, Salt and Blood Pressure, Substance abuse along with Exercise are areas within our control and can prevent or delay heart disease.

B. Managing our Time, Tongue, Priorities and Attitudes and Influence along with Exercising selflessness toward Godliness are areas within our control and will go a long way to promote personal and church growth.

5. **Stomp out Stress**

A. Seek First the kingdom of God Mat 6:33-34, Mat 6:25 Luk 10:41-42
B. Under a Broom Tree? I Ki 19
C. Develop Healthy Relationships; Ecc 4:9-12, Pro 27:17, Pro. 17:17, Pro 18:24, Jam 5:16, Mat 21:21-22

6. **Realize that Less is More**

A. Junk Food
B. Eli's evil sons; I Sa 2:12 through 3:13 and I Sa 4:17-18, Judg 3:12-30
C. Substance Abuse. Pro 23:20-21, Eph 5:18-21, Pro 31:6-7, 1Ti 5:23

7. **Cruise Ship Living?**

A. Lifestyle, Healthy People 2010 Incentive/Medicare reform
B. Obesity
   1. Body Mass Index (BMI); Free App. From NIH Called BMI calculator
   2. Waist circumference >35 inches in the non-pregnant
C. Tools to help:
   1. MyFitnessPal free app.
   2. ChooseMYPLATE.gov

8. **Pass the Salt**

A. Influence; Mat 5:13, Gal 5:9
B. Traded for Gold, Col 4:6
C. Saving aspects, 2 Ch 13:5
D. Daniel and Friends, Dan 1:3-21, Mat 10:28

E. Coffee Bean story pg. 119 in Heart and Soul

9. **Tame the Tongue**
   A. The Tongue, Rom 16:17-18, Jam 3:5-6, Jam 3:13,
   B. Going Viral, Pro 18:8
   C. Ambassadors, Pro 4:23-24, Pro 32:4
   D. Toxic, Pro 28:10, Pro 20:17
   E. The mouth speaks from the Abundance of the Heart, Mat 12:33-37, Pro18:21
   F. It's Tricky, Ecc 3:7

10. **Choose this Fruit**
   A. Super Foods Fight Cancer-Antioxidants
   B. Spiritual Antioxidants, Pro 11:30,
   Known by our Fruit, Gal 5:22-23

11. **Limit the Sweets**
   A. Eat what is Sufficient, Pro 25:16
   B. Sweeter than Honey, Psa 119:103-104
   C. Eat More Whole Grains
   D. Manna from Above, Jn 6:31-33
   E. Living Bread, Jn 6:35, Jn 6:51

12. **Heart Healthy Essentials**
   A. Don't Forget the Dairy, I Pe 2:1-3
   B. Desire Solid Food, Heb 5:13-14
   C. Douse the Flames! (Managing our Anger) Pro 16: 32, 6:32 Pro 15:18, Pro 15:1, Mat 5:9, Col 3:8, Ecc 7:9
   D. Hydrate Hydrate Hydrate! 1Pe 3:18-22. Gen 6:13, Heb.11:7

13. **Setting Priorities**
   A. Meat for the Belly, I Co 6:13
   B. Treasures, Mat 6:21, Pro 23:23
   C. Reflections. What do we reflect to God and others?
   D. Throw out the Bitter Spices, Jam 3:14-18
   Put First Things First, Jn 6:27, Eph 1:13-14

14. **Choose this Fruit**

A. Setting Spiritual Goals

Make a S.M.A.R.T. goal. Specific, Measurable, Action oriented, Realistic within a specific Time frame. For example, instead of saying, "I want to be more compassionate", Say "I want to call all the people on our sick list. Have a sister over that is struggling in some way, for coffee. Send a card to the new converts, walk over and meet the new neighbors this week."

B. Pick a Fruit of the Month, Gal 5:22-23

C. Have a Positive Attitude! Phi. 4:11-13

15. **Practice Selflessness**

A. The Importance of Strength Training

B. Bear One Another's' Burdens; Gal 6:2-3

C. Geese story pg. 66 Heart and Soul

D. Exercise Selflessness, Phi 2:3

E. Nourish your Body, Eph 5:29

F. Exercise toward Godliness,1 Co 9:224-7, 1 Ti 4:7-8

1. Digging Deeper online studies with Cindy Colley
2. Missions, Consider behind the scenes work
3. Disaster Relief
4. Teach World Bible School Online Bible correspondence classes
5. Teach World English Institute

16. **Conditioning the Core**

A. Importance of core exercises.

B. Strength to Your Flesh, Pro 3:5-8

C. Pro 3:5-8 (KJV) and (ASV) reads "Health to your navel and marrow to your bones." Navel is the connection site for the umbilical cord. Marrow is the Core of blood cell formation. Strong's uses the word "refreshment" for marrow. Can't get more Core than this!

D. NO Accident that we cannot live without Water and Blood physically or spiritually, Mar 16:16, Rom 3:25-26, Rom 5:9, Gal 3:27, 1 Pe 3:18-22

E. Listen to The Great Physician, Follow the treatment plan and Take your medicine!

- Please remember before starting any new nutrition or exercise plan to check with your physician. Please feel free to contact me if you have questions about anything that was said. I love to hear about your success stories any time. I am on Facebook using my maiden name and married name due to other authors with the same name. Please friend or message me anytime at Karen Hall Thompson or email at kjthompson60@gmail.com
If I can help in any way.

have saved someone's kidneys and the need for dialysis, I am greatly saddened.

We can let the little incidents with people at work, at home, or in the church burden us down and drive our blood pressure up. I have heard of ladies who argue and squabble about who will make the cookies for Vacation Bible School. This behavior describes the words *hyper* and *tension*! Left unchecked, it will split the church.

Worries and Troubles

Martha was consumed with the little things of life. She wanted Jesus to make her sister Mary help her prepare for guests, but Mary wanted to sit at Jesus' feet and listen to Him. Jesus said, "Martha, Martha, you are worried and troubled about many things. But one thing is needed, and Mary has chosen that good part" (Luke 10:41–42). Mary understood what was important. She did not sweat the small things. She filled her life with Jesus.

The late sister Jane McWhorter held many ladies day events for our congregation. I heard her state, "Before my first car accident—in 1970 when I was 35—I worked myself crazy every time I tried to entertain or prepare for a fellowship meal. I cooked and cleaned and scrubbed, preparing to the point I could not enjoy my guests or participate in the discussion or fun." That terrible disfiguring car accident taught her what was important in life. Jane would say, "I learned to give myself a KISS when entertaining: Keep it simple, stupid." What wonderful advice! Let's learn to enjoy each other's company, help each other get to heaven, and not get so caught up in the trivialities of decorations or food preparation.

Heart and Soul

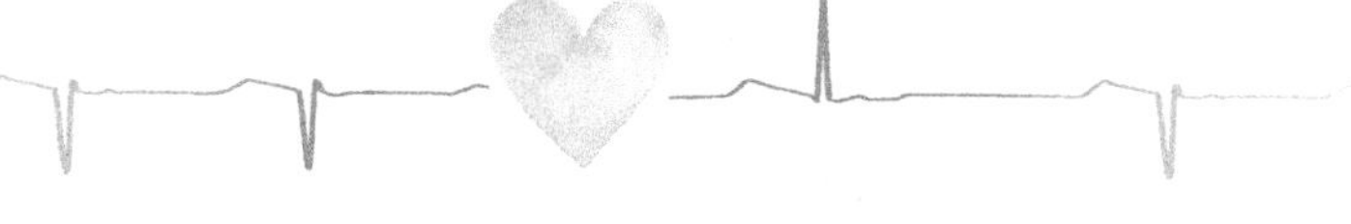

"Set your mind on things above, not on things on the earth" (Colossians 3:2).

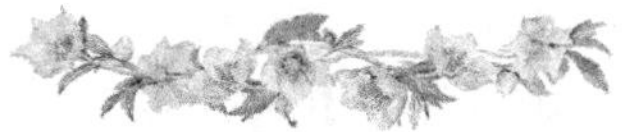

Uncontrolled blood pressure can weaken your heart and put you at risk for heart failure. A heart in failure does not snap back to fill or squeeze and do the work it did before. I am convinced that discouraged Christian women can allow unhealthy communications and relationships with family members, co-workers, or close friends weaken her physical and spiritual heart. She is carrying too much weight and living under too much pressure. And often she does not snap back.

Recovery is slow and painful after a heart attack or stroke. Christians are affected daily. Take charge of your life. Manage your risk factors. God needs healthy workers. Remember, heart disease is the number one killer of men *and* women. Getting these numbers in control will go a long way to getting you back on the road to physical health so you can do the Lord's work.

Warm-Ups

Invite a health-care worker to class to take blood pressures and get weights and waist circumferences, or bring a scale and cloth tape measure to class and privately determine your own waist circumference and height. Determine what your ideal weight range would be based on the BMI (Body Mass Index) range. Use a BMI calculator app or use a BMI chart by NIH (National Institute of Health).

Soul Stretches

- Take a personal inventory of your spiritual burdens. How might you be enabling weakness in others by carrying too much weight yourself?
- Research scripture about bearing burdens—your own and those of others. Look for examples from characters such as Hezekiah (2 Kings 19–20) and David (Psalm 142:1–2).

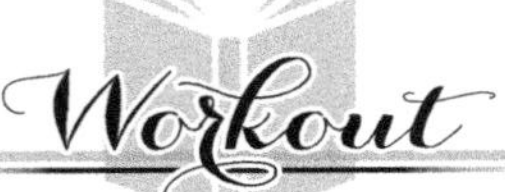

Workout

1. What is the biggest health risk facing the United States?

2. Is being overweight or obese the church's problem? Is uncontrolled high blood pressure the church's problem?

3. Read Daniel 1 and discuss how Daniel's food choices were a precursor to the DASH Diet.

4. Define *dialysis*. How can ignoring high blood pressure contribute to the need for dialysis?

5. When a discouraged Christian allows her spiritual weights to weaken her soul, she might not snap back. Who have you known in

that situation? What steps might prevent this heavy burden? How can you help?

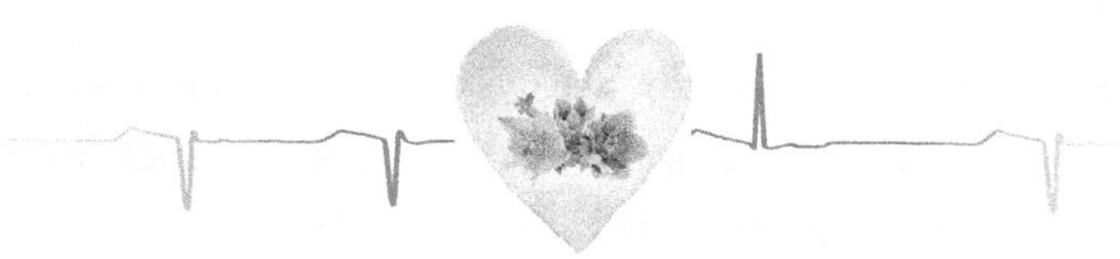

2

Eliminate Overindulgence

"Do not mix with winebibbers, or with gluttonous eaters of meat: for the drunkard and the glutton will come to poverty, and drowsiness will clothe a man with rags" (Proverbs 23:20–21).

How Much Is Enough?

Eating in excess and lusting after food or drink for self-gratification or emotional fulfillment is unhealthy physically, emotionally, and spiritually. It is important to understand why we eat or drink. Are we hungry or thirsty, or are we trying to fill a hole in our heart caused by loneliness or boredom? Have you ever gone through a buffet line and seen people pile food on their plates four to five inches high? Because of the large amount of blood it takes to digest your food, your heart has to work harder. This is why exercising right after a large meal is not generally recommended.

Do you think your body needs that much food? It may surprise you to learn that a serving of meat is roughly the size of a deck of cards. Would it also surprise you to learn a portion of whole grain breads, bagels, and rice is no bigger than the size of your fist? The app ChooseMyPlate.gov has great visual suggestions on how to make good portion choices. Portion control is critical to a healthy weight and healthy life. Think about how much money is spent eating out.

You must ask yourself, "How am I using the financial resources God has blessed me with? Am I eating or drinking my paycheck away? Am I making good choices about what I eat and put into my body?"

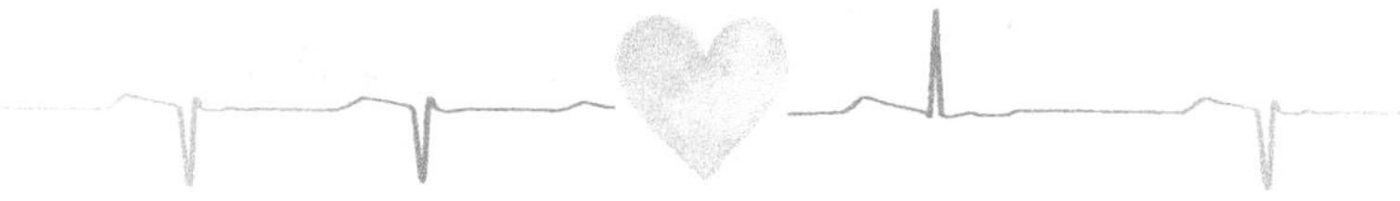

"My flesh and my heart fail; but God is the strength of my heart and my portion forever" (Psalm 73:26).

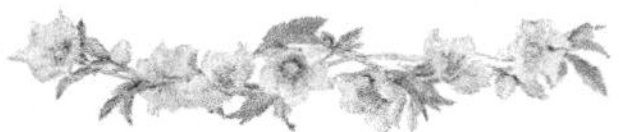

The Skinny on Fats

There is a great deal of confusion out there about fats. We must have fats to live. Fat is an insulator and is used to metabolize "fat soluble vitamins." Saturated fats are solid at room temperature: the visible fat on a steak, lamb, pork, poultry with skin, butter, cheese, cream cheese, lard, and solid vegetable shortening, such as Crisco. Too much fat, especially the saturated kind, is associated with an increase in cardiovascular clogging of the arteries.

Too many trans fats and partially hydrogenated vegetable oils are also believed to be unhealthy. Many snack and highly processed foods such as baked cookies and cakes, doughnuts, fried foods, refrigerator dough, creamer, and margarine, are loaded with this type of fat. We

all must read labels closely to avoid too much of the unhealthy type of fat.[13]

Too many saturated fats and trans fats can lead to an increase of plaque and "clogging" in your arteries. This is why we check cholesterol levels to evaluate risk. When someone has a fasting lipid panel to check her cholesterol, these are the values that are reviewed.

Here are the ABCs in discussing a cholesterol panel:

- LDL stands for low-density lipoproteins, the "lousy" part of your cholesterol panel. It needs to be low.
- HDL stands for high-density lipoproteins, the "healthy" part of your cholesterol panel. It needs to be high.
- TGL stands for triglycerides, the circulating fat.

Saturated and trans fats can increase the LDL. It is when the LDL is too high and the HDL is too low and TGL is too high that plaque becomes a problem.

What Is Cholesterol?

Cholesterol makes up bile acids used in the digestion of food and with vitamin D production, as well as hormones such as estrogen and testosterone. It also makes up the membranes of cells. It travels through the body in packages called lipoproteins. The inside of these packages is lipids or fat and the outside is a protein.[14]

The confusing thing is that cholesterol is not fat. It is a waxy substance that is produced mostly by your own liver and is necessary for life. To help my patients figure out which foods have cholesterol, I remind them that cholesterol is only found in animal products. Anything that had a liver or came from an animal with a liver, such as eggs, milk, and butter, contains cholesterol. It is not found in vegetable

products, so that's why a label on a can of Crisco can read "zero percent cholesterol" but be a hundred percent fat.

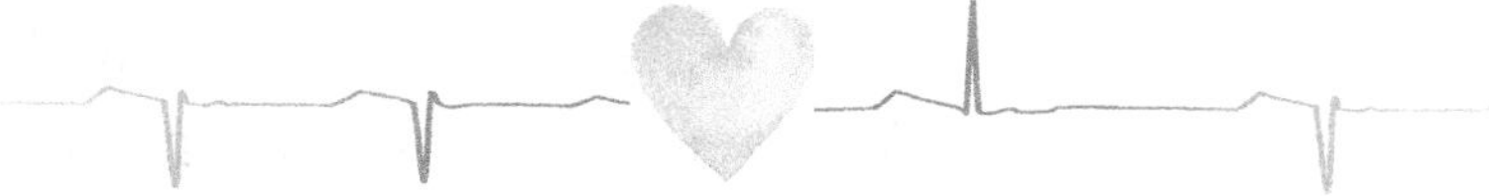

"And the priest shall burn them on the altar as food, an offering made by fire for a sweet aroma; all the fat is the Lord's. This shall be a perpetual statute throughout your generations in all your dwellings: you shall eat neither fat nor blood" (Leviticus 3:16–17).

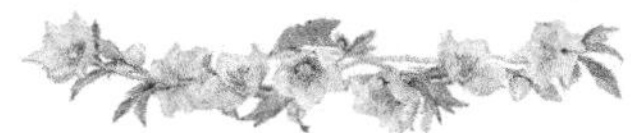

Eat It Today and Wear It Tomorrow

Junk food is not nutritious in any way. It has excess calories, too much fat, too much salt, and too much sugar that slow us down. Ladies, Satan is trying to use our wealthy and sedentary me-focused lifestyles against us, making us too fat and too tired to do God's work. That old saying is true: Eat it today and wear it tomorrow. Our metabolism is believed to slow with the aging process, and that extra weight seems to "mold to our bones" and become more and more difficult to get rid of.

How many times have you gone to McDonald's and ordered a Big Mac meal? If you include an apple pie with it, you consume 1,480 calories in one meal which contains almost a whole day's worth of calories and salt for most of us.

Even a "nice" restaurant may illustrate the point of excess. Applebee's Appetizer Sampler contains more than two full days' worth of salt and 2,370 calories. Granted, this dish is an appetizer and meant to

be shared with others. But do not claim ignorance and ignore the facts. Buyer beware![15]

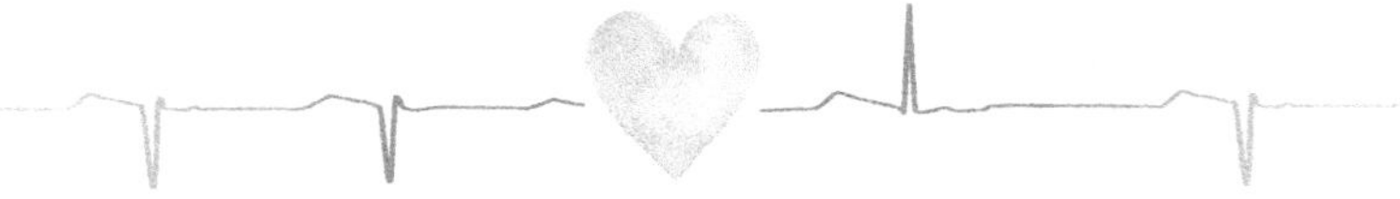

"There is a way that seems right to a man, but its end is the way of death" (Proverbs 14:12).

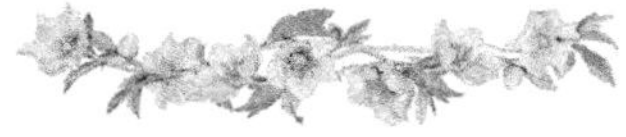

One Little M&M

Okay, so you'll eat a hot dog or pizza at home and have a few M&Ms instead of apple pie for dessert. When you realize how much exercise it takes to burn off these calories, you might change your mind:

- One hot dog requires 28 minutes of jogging at 5 miles per hour.
- A 12-inch pizza takes 117 minutes of aerobics.
- One M&M candy requires a walk the length of a football field.[16]

Too many calories, fat, and sugar can lead to obesity. It is no wonder we can put on weight so quickly.

Excess and too many self-indulgences and "treats" can lead to obesity. Obesity can lead to early activity limitations, serious health issues, and early death. Thyroid issues and other medical or orthopedic or neurological health problems make optimal weight difficult, but most of the time, obesity is the result of the choices we make.

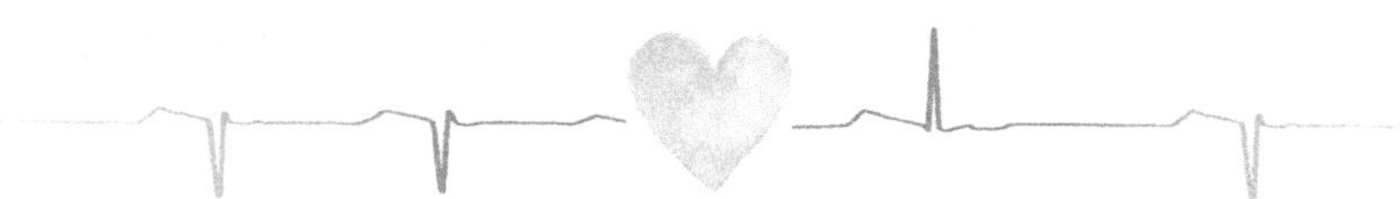

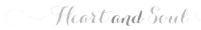

"Do not be deceived, God is not mocked; for whatever a man sows, that he will also reap. For he who sows to his flesh will of the flesh reap corruption, but he who sows to the Spirit will of the Spirit reap everlasting life" (Galatians 6:7–8).

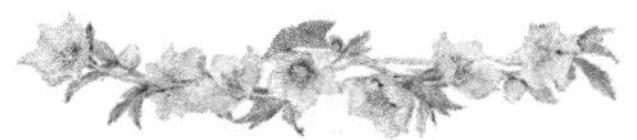

Lust to the Max

Barney Fife, a character on *The Andy Griffith Show*, would say the following story is an example of "ill-gotten gain."

Eli the priest had two evil sons, Hophni and Phinehas, who were also priests (1 Samuel 2:34). They lusted for the fatty portions of the meat that the men of Israel brought to the tabernacle. The fat was meant to be a sacrifice to the Lord, but Hophni and Phinehas demanded the raw meat with the fat that the worshipers brought. If the raw meat was not voluntarily surrendered, then Eli's sons took it by force. They also committed fornication with the women who assembled at the door of the tabernacle.

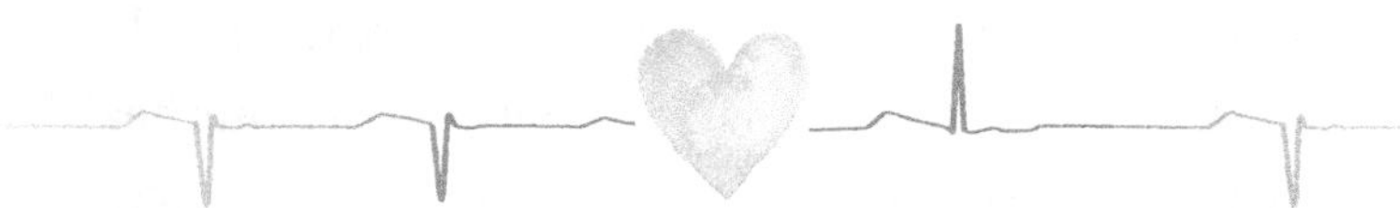

"Why do you kick at My sacrifice and My offering which I commanded in My dwelling place, and honor your sons more than Me, to make yourselves fat with the best of all the offerings of Israel My people?" (1 Samuel 2:29).

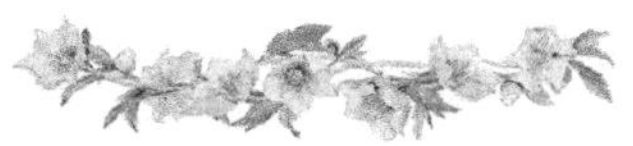

This is lust to the max. They were abusing their roles and the trust of the people and serving the Lord for their own selfish despicable gain. In 1 Samuel 2:23–24 Eli told his sons to stop this sinful behavior but they did not listen. In verses 27–29 a man of God came to Eli and said, "Why do you . . . make yourselves fat with the best of all the offerings of Israel My people?" God was not happy with Eli. He was accountable to God for his sons' despicable behavior because he did not restrain them.

The man of God told Eli that soon he would no longer be the priest and that all his descendants would die in the flower of their age because of his sons' sin and his own lack of restraint and discipline. The sign would be that his sons Hophni and Phinehas would die on the same day (1 Samuel 2:33–34).

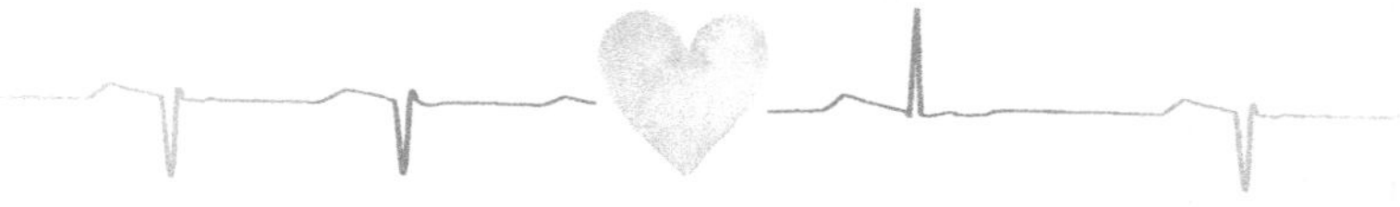

"Then it happened, when he made mention of the ark of God, that Eli fell off the seat backward by the side of the gate; and his neck was broken and he died, for the man was old and heavy" (1 Samuel 4:18).

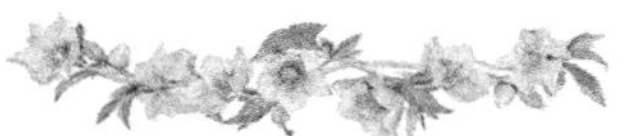

As Paul Harvey used to say, "Now the rest of the story." In 1 Samuel 4:7–18 we read that Hophni and Phinehas were killed by the Philistines, both on the same day, just as God had promised. It was the same day that the Ark of the Covenant was taken. Eli was greatly grieved about the deaths of his sons, but the real tragedy was that the Philistines had taken God's holy instrument, the Ark of the Covenant.

You can't help but wonder about Eli. Scripture relates that he was old and heavy. Was he partaking of this unbridled lust of the fatty meat

just like his sons? It appears so. Their actions had spiritual and physical consequences.

Ehud and Eglon

Judges 3 records an account of God's delivering His people into the hands of a pagan king because they did evil in His sight. Eglon captured them and held them for 18 years.

> The children of Israel again did evil in the sight of the Lord. So the Lord strengthened Eglon king of Moab against Israel, because they had done evil in the sight of the Lord. Then he gathered to himself the people of Ammon and Amalek, went and defeated Israel, and took possession of the City of Palms. So the children of Israel served Eglon king of Moab eighteen years (Judges 3:12–14).

God raised up a deliverer in Israel when they cried out to Him—Ehud, a left-handed man from the tribe of Benjamin. He was responsible for presenting tributes in the form of tax moneys to King Eglon of Moab. One day he took more than the tax collection; he crafted a double-edged dagger a cubit long and hid it under his clothes on his right thigh.

A cubit is 18 inches and the hilt or handle of a sword was probably six inches. So Ehud sent the others away and went to Eglon in his cool private chamber and tricked him into believing he had a secret message from God in order to get him alone. Then left-handed Ehud grabbed the dagger from his right thigh and thrust all 18 inches straight into Eglon's belly where it was immediately hidden in the fat, killing the king of Moab.

The description of the fat closing over the whole sword, including the handle, is morbid and distasteful. We can surmise that Eglon lived a life of excess likely at the expense of the children of Israel and was indeed clearly a very fat man. Fat seems to accompany excess.

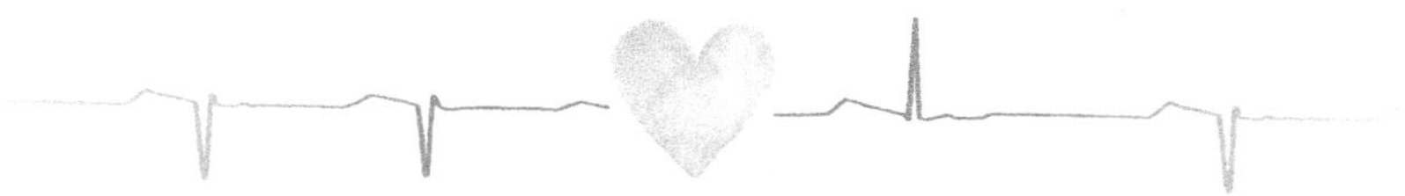

"Then Ehud said, 'I have a message from God for you.' So he [Eglon] arose from his seat. Then Ehud reached with his left hand, took the dagger from his right thigh, and thrust it into his belly. Even the hilt went in after the blade, and the fat closed over the blade, for he did not draw the dagger out of his belly; and his entrails came out" (Judges 3:20–22).

Super Bowl Sunday Secret

Fatty foods are not the only excess we should cut. Ninety billion dollars in W2 earnings and 400 billion in economic activity were associated with alcohol in the United States in 2010.[17]

I once visited my sister in downtown Chicago and there were people lying on the middle of the sidewalks in broad daylight with alcoholic beverages in their hands and dressed in dirty clothes that were torn. I wonder if Solomon had seen similar sights.

Alcohol impairs your thinking, lowers your inhibitions, and sets you up for failure personally and professionally. It can cost you your life or the lives of others.[18] You cannot predict how much it takes to impair you, and that is information you don't see in a beer commercial on Super Bowl Sunday.

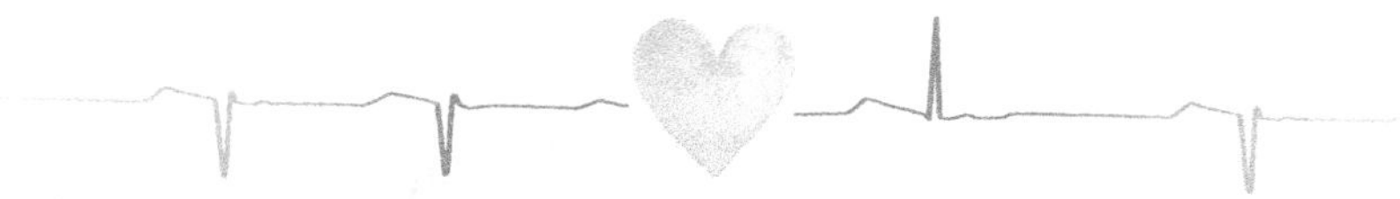

"For the drunkard and the glutton will come to poverty, and drowsiness will clothe a man with rags" (Proverbs 23:21).

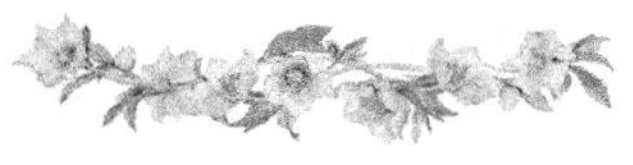

Be Wary of Research

Often my patients will say, "Karen, there was a study done in France that a drink of red wine every day is good for your heart." If I made parachutes for a living, I would devise a study that could prove that sky divers live longer if they wear a parachute when they jump from an airplane. Would that mean we all need to buy a parachute? All that to say, be careful with research, and know who is financially behind its published results.

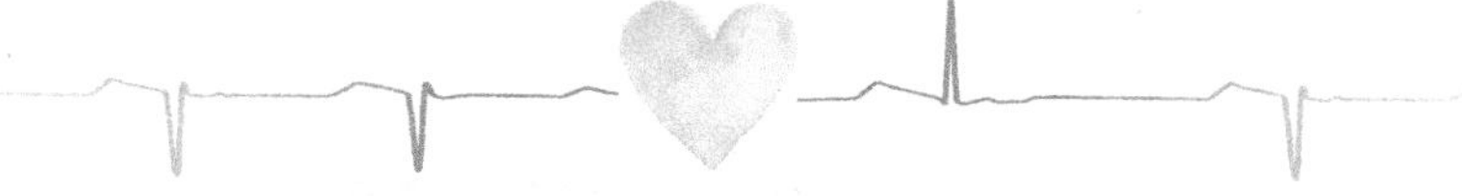

"Wine is a mocker, strong drink is a brawler, and whoever is led astray by it is not wise" (Proverbs 20:1).

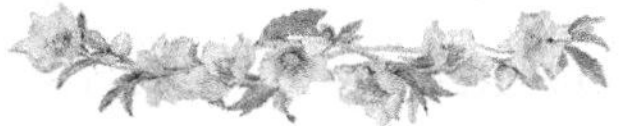

Dependence on alcohol can dull the senses and weaken the heart. There is no evidence that a non-drinker should start drinking for health benefits. There is much evidence that the flavonoids that give the grape its color provide the health benefits rather than the alcohol. Flavonoids are often found in the colorful pigment of plants and are believed to provide many health benefits including inflammation control, useful with allergies, cell structure protection due to the antioxidant effect, and vitamin C support.[19]

Do You Need Alcohol?

Paul says: "Do not be drunk with wine, in which is dissipation [excess]; but be filled with the Spirit" (Ephesians 5:18). When Paul says, be filled with the Spirit, he uses *pneuma* for "Spirit." He is saying, be filled with God, just as you fill your lungs with air. Fill your life with godly things.

If a woman says she needs alcohol to feel good, does she have a problem? Could she be trying to mask the true problem or fill an emptiness or hole in her heart? Are some people today trying to anesthetize themselves by using alcohol?

TV shows try to make alcohol look sophisticated and cool, as they did cigarettes years ago. Remember the Marlboro man? The tobacco ads featured robust, healthy, handsome cowboys smoking. Ironically, five of the actors who appeared in these ads died of lung cancer or other smoking-related disease complications.[20] Please do not be deceived by the marketers and sponsors of TV shows.

A Mayo Clinic article advised that chronic alcoholism can cause liver damage. The liver makes vital nutrients and acts as a filter and detoxifies and cleans harmful substances from your body. Cirrhosis happens when scar tissue is formed to repair this injury. This type of damage can be treated but generally cannot be undone.[21] Long-term alcohol abuse weakens and thins the heart muscle and can raise blood pressure. The weakened heart cannot pump blood as it once did, so the user's vital organs are deprived of oxygenated blood.[22]

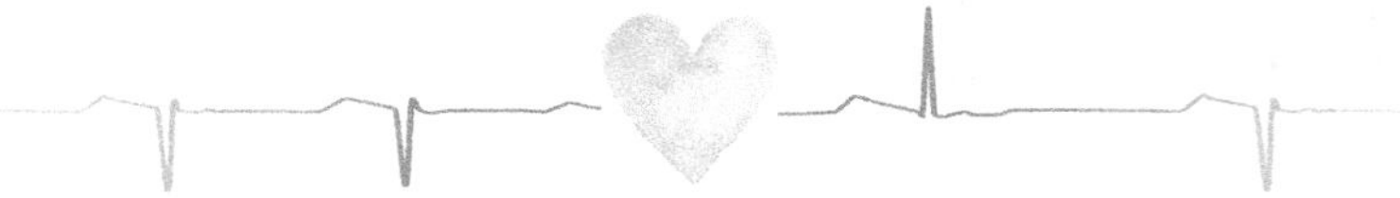

"But each one is tempted when he is carried away and enticed by his own lust" (James 1:14).

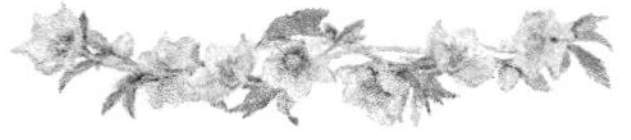

Under Social Influence

Some say, "I just drink for social reasons." Even one drink can impair judgment and slow reaction time. In 2012, 10,322 people were killed because of alcohol-impaired driving. Twenty percent of the deaths

were children 14 years old and under.[23] Think about the social implications of impaired drinking. What if you were the driver in an accident that resulted in the death of a child? I encourage you not to drink for social reasons. There is a relatively new slogan on TV to discourage impaired driving: "Buzzed driving is drunk driving." How true!

Jesus' first recorded miracle of changing water to wine (John 2:1–11) is frequently cited as reason enough to drink socially. Nothing about Jesus' actions corroborate His approval of drunkenness or getting "buzzed." Would you be comfortable if Jesus attended your tailgate party? Would He want to attend?

Proverbs 31:6 states, "Give strong drink to him who is perishing, and wine to those who are bitter of heart." First Timothy 5:23 reads, "No longer drink only water, but use a little wine for your stomach's sake and your frequent infirmities." These biblical citations demonstrate that alcohol is not used to strengthen an individual, or to aid in their productivity, or to promote clearer thinking either in society or in the Lord's church. Rather, these citations illustrate that alcohol is not used to become strong but for those with an infirmity. Sisters, this is not popular. The Lord's church does not need people under the influence. The Lord's church needs men and women and children who do the influencing.

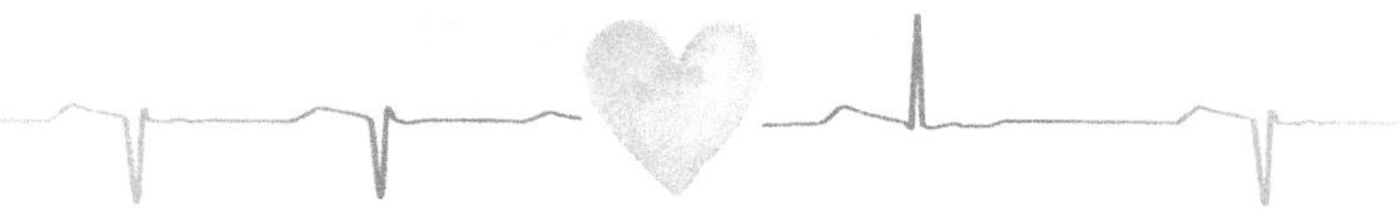

"So it is not the will of your Father who is in heaven that one of these little ones perish" (Matthew 18:14).

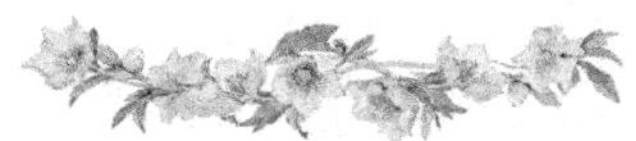

Deceit of Narcotics

When I was a new nurse working the 3–11 PM shift, a patient was admitted right at the change of shift. While I was giving a report to the new shift, a patient put on her emergency bathroom call bell, and we found her on the floor. We discovered a large stone in the urine collection "hat" in the toilet, collected it, and sent it to the lab.

We called the "stat" team to evaluate and x-ray her for other kidney stones and fall injuries. I stayed and called the physician, and he prescribed intravenous morphine for pain relief. I was very late getting home that night but happy that this woman was out of pain. When I got back to work the next day, she had been discharged. The lab report revealed that the stone collected was a piece of gravel from outside and that there were other "stones" taped to her body to appear as if they were in her kidneys. Why? Intravenous morphine. She was craving the opioid morphine so much she went to this extreme.

Prescription drugs, especially the opioid variety, marijuana, and illegal street drugs have addictive tendencies. Good people can accidentally get hooked after an injury before they realize it. I once knew someone who carried her prescription narcotics in the jewelry she wore for easy access. She called them her "happy pills." Her family said she would set the clock so she would remember to take her medicine every four hours. They would have to arrange their vacation time around access and refill times of the drug. She noticed that it kept taking more and more of the drug to ease her pain. In further conversation, she admitted she was taking the pills to prevent the pain from returning rather than using them to relieve pain. This is part of the deceiving qualities of narcotics that can actually drive a need and subsequent addiction.

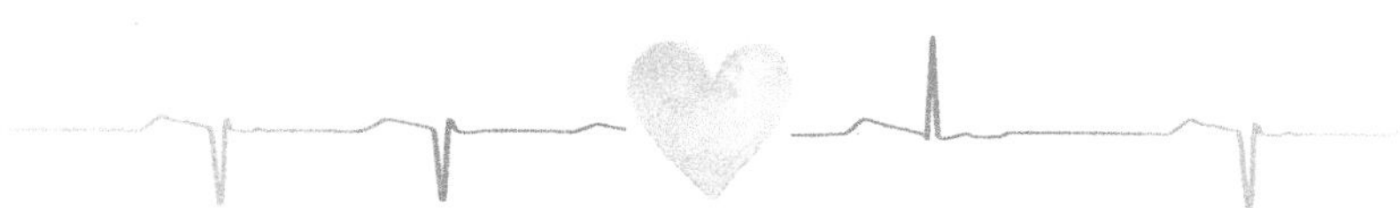

"Do you not know that the unrighteous will not inherit the kingdom of God? Do not be deceived. Neither fornicators, nor idolaters, nor adulterers, nor homosexuals, nor sodomites, nor thieves, nor covetous, nor drunkards, nor revilers, nor extortioners will inherit the kingdom of God. And such were some of you. But you were washed, but you were sanctified, but you were justified in the name of the Lord Jesus and by the Spirit of our God" (1 Corinthians 6:9–11).

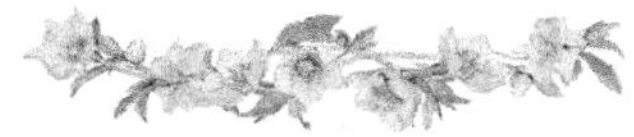

Prescription for Prevention

Alcohol and drugs are known to lower inhibitions. In other words, people of all ages under their influence remove clothing, say inappropriate things, do inappropriate things, have illicit sexual encounters, have slower reaction times, and experience impaired memories and judgment. My patients have shared with me that often their thinking is so cloudy after drinking or using one of these substances that they have no memory of their actions afterward. Consequences include unwanted pregnancies, dismemberment, job loss and financial ruin, ruined relationships, and even death. Many a tear has been shed over the associated guilt and shame and hurt caused to others, especially innocent victims. These consequences cannot be undone. What is the answer?

My dad sells real estate and has told us the three most important things to remember about real estate buying and selling are "Location. Location. Location." In health care the three most important things to remember are "Prevention. Prevention. Prevention." People say to me,

"Well, my doctor prescribed it. It is legal. I need it. I can't get through the day without it." What is the root of the problem? Is it really the pain driving the need for the medicine or is there an underlying emotional issue driving the need to mask the pain? Pull off the mask and do some soul searching.

Warning: Don't taste, touch, or handle addictive substances! If deemed necessary, use for only the shortest amount of time possible. The deaths of Elvis Presley, Michael Jackson, and Prince have shined a spotlight on the physical, emotional, and yes, spiritual problems associated with their alleged legal prescription drug and substance abuse. Satan wins when he can impair, influence, and distract us from doing God's will.

There are many who will beg, steal, and scam money from good people in order to buy drugs and alcohol. This behavior often leads to unemployment and poverty or worse, jail or death. I have often seen mothers, fathers, and grandparents making excuses for, or enabling their loved ones inadvertently. Pray for God's assistance, enlist the help of the church, and seek professional assistance to break the chains of addiction.

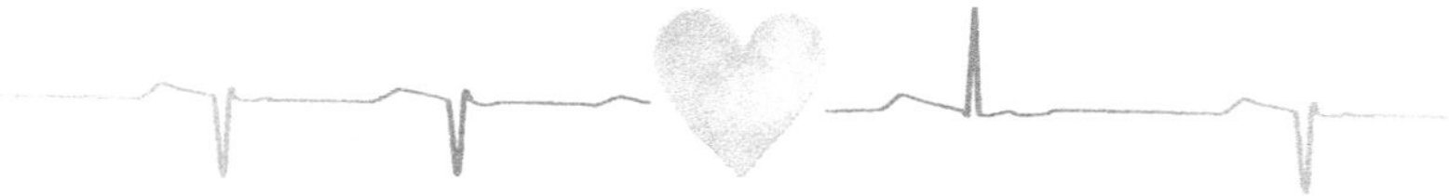

"No temptation has overtaken you except such as is common to man; but God is faithful, who will not allow you to be tempted beyond what you are able, but with the temptation will also make the way of escape, that you may be able to bear it" (1 Corinthians 10:13).

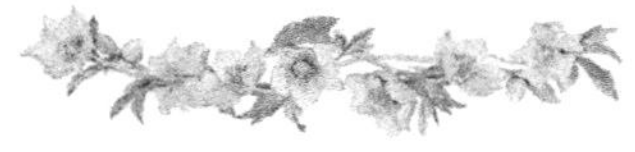

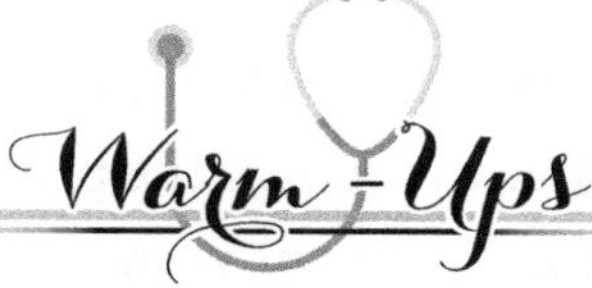

Warm-Ups

- Share how alcohol and/or legal or illegal drugs or substances have impacted your life or a loved one's life, physically and spiritually. What did it take to overcome the addiction?
- Research resources in your hometown that deal with addictions.

Soul Stretches

Do a Bible word search on *wine* and pray that God will give you an open mind. Make notes of your findings, and then answer these thought-provoking questions:

1. Am I a better person when I drink?
2. Are my children better when I drink?
3. Does the United States need teachers, school bus drivers, doctors, nurses, pilots, truck drivers, employees, employers, children, retirees, judges, juries, and leaders who are impaired by drugs?
4. Does alcohol make me a better ambassador for the kingdom of God?
5. Does the Lord's church need men and women or children, "under the influence"?

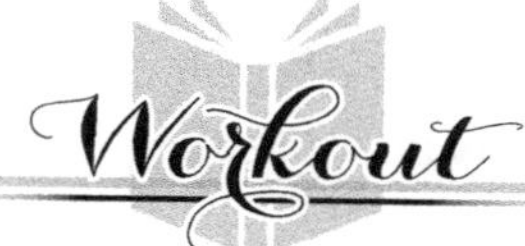

❶ Look closely at the nutrition label on your favorite "healthy" food. What percentage of saturated and trans fats does it contain? Were you surprised?

---

❷ What is an easy way to remember the types of foods that contain cholesterol?

---

❸ What were the consequences of the actions of Eli's corrupt sons (1 Samuel 4:7–18)?

---

❹ What were the short-term and long-term repercussions of the deaths of Eli, Hophni, and Phinehas to their families and those around them (1 Samuel 2:33–34)?

---

❺ How might one blame the Bible or American Heart Association or Center for Disease Control for his own lack of self-control in handling addiction?

---

❻ Read and discuss Ephesians 5:18.

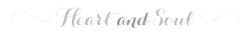

7. Discuss Jesus' changing water to wine in John 2:1–11. Does that mean social drinking is acceptable to God? Support your answer.

8. Why is dependence on substances such as drugs and alcohol a problem for the church?

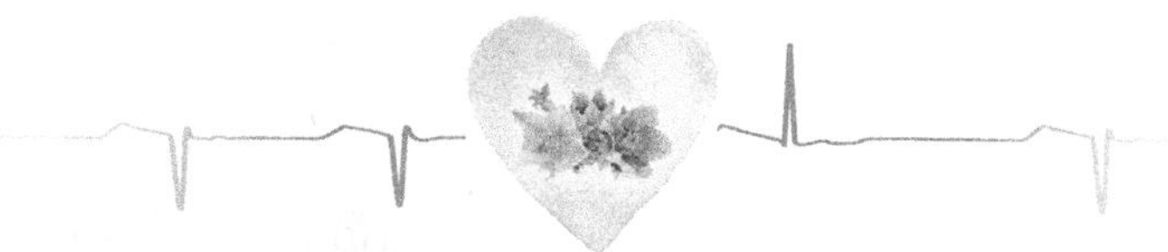

—3—

Choose This Fruit

But the fruit of the Spirit is love, joy, peace, longsuffering, kindness, goodness, faithfulness, gentleness, self-control. Against such there is no law (Galatians 5:22–23).

As a joke, we bought our adult son one-piece Superman pajamas. Now he is known as "Super Daddy," and he and his family occasionally dress up as super heroes and fight off the "bad guys" to protect the world.

I like to imagine the nutrients in fruits and vegetables fighting off the "bad guys" in our bodies at the cellular level. These "super foods" fight off the free radicals and oxidant "bad guys" to protect our body from harm.

Antioxidants (also known as super foods) are a hot topic these days. Here are a few reasons:

- Antioxidants, such as cranberries and blueberries, are believed to possess protective health benefits.[24]
- The antioxidant effects of fresh fruits and veggies are believed to be cancer fighting.
- Antioxidant vitamins, vitamin C for example, are believed to remove free radicals or damaging oxidizing agents from our bodies.

In 2012, I attended the National American Association of Cardiovascular and Pulmonary Rehab Conference in Orlando, Florida. The dietician who spoke that day suggested using a color method to improve nutrition. She suggested five colors on a plate as being "healthy." For example, a nutritional value point would be assigned for each color: one green plus one red plus one purple should equal three points. But according to the dietician at the conference, they may actually equal six points instead because of the multiplying vitamin effect. This is an interesting theory about how colorful foods when combined may enhance the nutritional value of the entire plate. However, there is very little, if any research, to corroborate that theory at this time.

It is still recommended today to eat a variety of colorful fruits and vegetables. Colors often represent an associated nutrient and phytochemical. For example, the anthocyanins are associated with blueberries and are what make the blueberry blue. It is the phytochemicals and flavonoids that are believed to be the heart-healthy and cancer-fighting antioxidants. ChooseMyPlate.gov suggests filling half your plate with fruits and vegetables, with vegetables being the larger section.

So put good, pure, fresh fruit and vegetables on your plate. There is nothing more delicious to me than a bowl of fresh blueberries or strawberries. Fresh foods, in general, are considered more nutritional than frozen. But frozen foods are more nutritional than canned because many nutrients are lost during the cooking and preserving process.

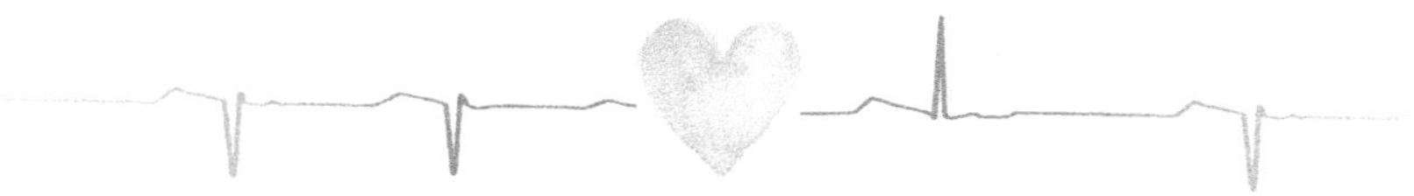

"Say to the righteous that it shall be well with them, for they shall eat the fruit of their doings" (Isaiah 3:10).

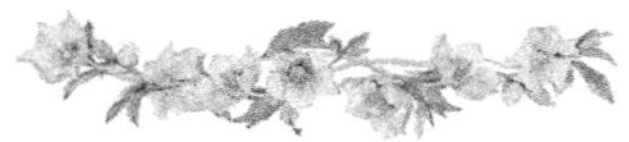

No Law against Spiritual Fruit

We should also load up on the fruit of the Spirit to promote spiritual health, not only for ourselves but also for those around us. "But the fruit of the Spirit is love, joy, peace, longsuffering, kindness, goodness, faithfulness, gentleness, self-control. Against such there is no law" (Galatians 5:22–23).

Against such there is no law? That is truly amazing. Do you know how many laws are on the book in our nation? There are 20,000 on gun control alone. The IRS code contains 3.4 million words, and if printed 60 lines per page, it would be 7,500 pages long.[25]

There are 613 laws in the Talmud, a collection of writings on Jewish law and custom and religious practice. How many federal laws do we have? No one knows. How many laws are there in the world? No one knows. But in all those laws, this passage says there is no law against love, joy, peace, longsuffering, kindness, goodness, faithfulness, gentleness, and self-control.

If we do a word study from *Strong's Dictionary* on the fruit of the Spirit, we can easily see why there is no law against them. Note the meanings of the names for words that comprise the fruit of the Spirit:

- *Love* [ἀγάπη agapē]—benevolence, affection, and charity.
- *Joy* [χαρά chara]—cheerfulness and gladness.

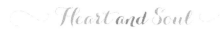

- *Peace* [εἰρήνη eirēnē]—prosperity, quietness, rest, and harmony.
- *Longsuffering* [μακροθυμία makrothymia]—fortitude, forbearance, patience, steadfastness, perseverance, and slowness in avenging wrong.
- *Kindness* [χρηστότης chrēstotēs]—usefulness, moral excellence, gentleness, moral integrity.
- *Goodness* [ἀγαθωσύνη agathōsynē]—virtue, uprightness of heart and life.
- *Faithfulness* [πίστις pistis]—moral conviction, belief, assurance, and fidelity.
- *Gentleness* [πρᾳότης praotēs]—humility, mildness, and meekness.
- *Self-control* [ἐγκράτεια egkrateia]—temperance, masters one's desires and passions, especially sensual appetites.

A righteous and godly person must possess these characteristics. It is sweet and comforting to be surrounded by loving Christian brothers and sisters who exhibit these characteristics, especially in times of trouble.

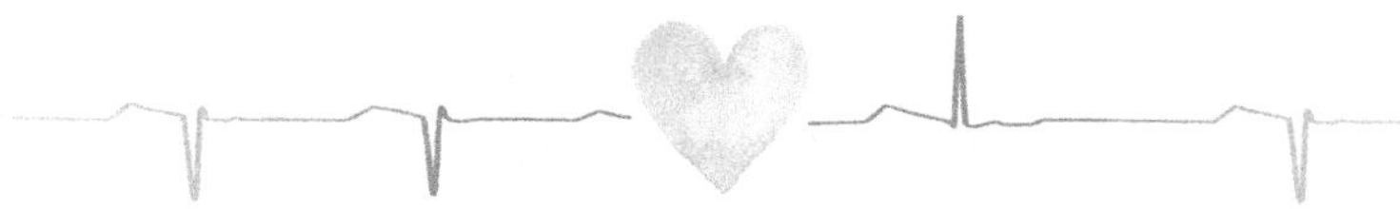

"Either make the tree good and its fruit good, or else make the tree bad and its fruit bad; for a tree is known by its fruit. Brood of vipers! How can you, being evil, speak good things? For out of the abundance of the heart the mouth speaks" (Matthew 12:33–34).

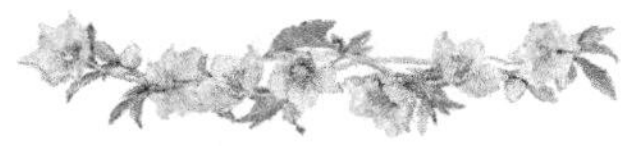

What Kind of Fruit Are You?

Jesus said, "A tree is known by its fruit." People will know if we are a good tree or a bad one by what we say and do—by the "fruit" we bear. Never once did my dad plant an apple tree that produced oranges.

Jesus knew what was in the Pharisees' hearts just as He knows what is in our hearts (Matthew 12:33–34). What is in our hearts will bubble up to the surface. Eventually our motives will be seen by our actions. In other words, our hearts will tell on us. It is hard to hide what we are really thinking or doing. Others can see right through us. Matthew says, "For where your treasure is, there your heart will be also" (Matthew 6:21).

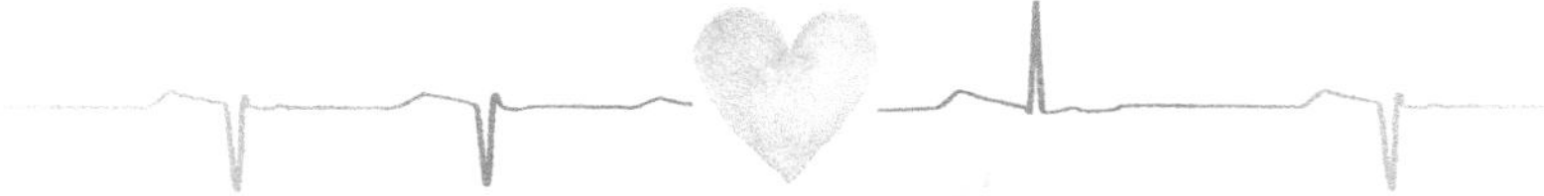

"For you were once darkness, but now you are light in the Lord. Walk as children of light (for the fruit of the Spirit is in all goodness, righteousness, and truth), finding out what is acceptable to the Lord" (Ephesians 5:8–10).

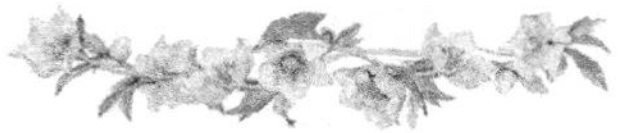

Be Genuine; Love More

James encourages us to be genuine in our Christian walk. If you want to be more loving, then invite people to your home, and be a hugger and a greeter at church and at home. Give freely of your time and money to the needy who are all around you, doing all in the name of the Lord. The only thing worse than being called a hypocrite is actually being a hypocrite. If your only job at church is to warm a pew on Sunday morning, maybe it is time to reevaluate your career choice.

Paul teaches us we must put on the tender mercies of kindness, humility, meekness, and longsuffering, but most of all love.

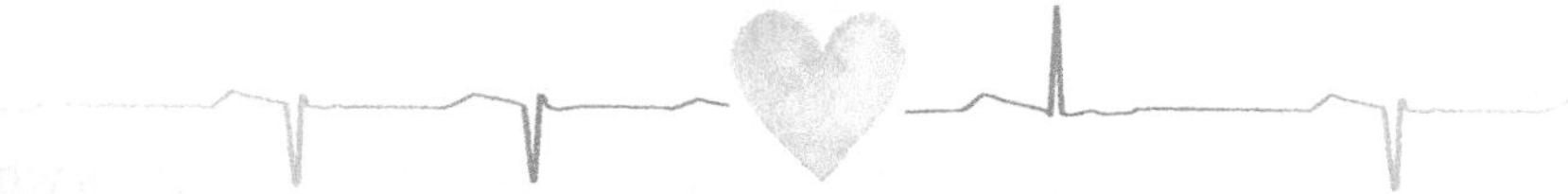

"Therefore, as the elect of God, holy and beloved, put on tender mercies, kindness, humility, meekness, longsuffering; bearing with one another, and forgiving one another, if anyone has a complaint against another; even as Christ forgave you, so you also must do. But above all these things put on love, which is the bond of perfection" (Colossians 3:12–14).

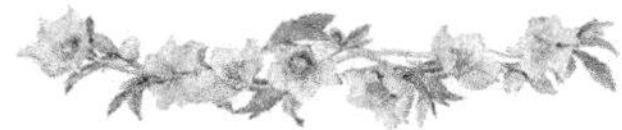

If you want to have more joy and be more joyful, then adopt cheerful and glad attitudes in all you set out to do, and smile at everyone. People will often reflect the expression you have on your face as you pass by in the hallway unless they have something else on their minds. Do not assume their expression is directed at you. Follow up with them and ask, "Are you okay? You seemed a little sad this afternoon." You may be surprised at their response. Letting them know you noticed shows you care.

In Proverbs 11:30, Solomon says, "The fruit of the righteous is a tree of life, and he who wins souls is wise." What does that mean? This imagery seems to imply that the righteous are active and living and interested in bearing spiritual fruit. Be fruity—spiritually speaking!

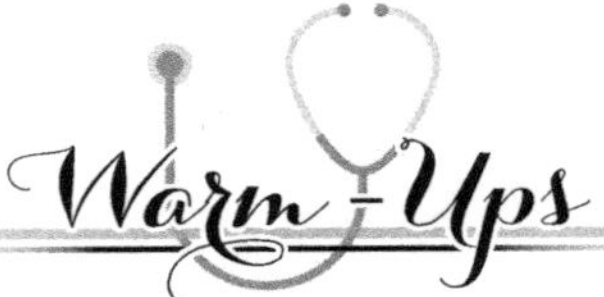

Warm-Ups

Challenge a sister to order a pizza and have it delivered while you make salad with grilled chicken on top. Compare the actual cost per person and then also compare the actual time it took to be put on your table. You may be very surprised. Now for fun look up the fat, protein, and carbohydrate content of the pizza compared to the salad. Discuss which one is the better buy.

Soul Stretches

- Without looking up Galatians 5:22–23, write down the fruit of the Spirit. If you missed one or two, make it your goal to memorize the entire list this week. Consider assigning each fruit a name that corresponds with its first letter or color of the fruit. For example, you could cut out or draw a kiwi and name it Kitty for Kindness and so on.
- Share some ways you or a loved one were "fruity" today.

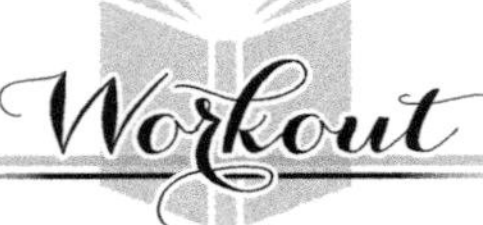

Workout

❶ What actions will you take to promote peace in the home or in the church or at the workplace?

❷ How will you be more patient, kind, faithful, good, and gentle?

---

❸ What is your plan to practice more self-control?

---

❹ Compare truth, candor, and genuineness to hypocrisy in our Christian walk.

---

❺ Seek out one individual in the church who appears sad, distant, or angry, and reach out to her in kindness. Take her a bowl of fresh strawberries, write her a note, or show some other small act of kindness.

4

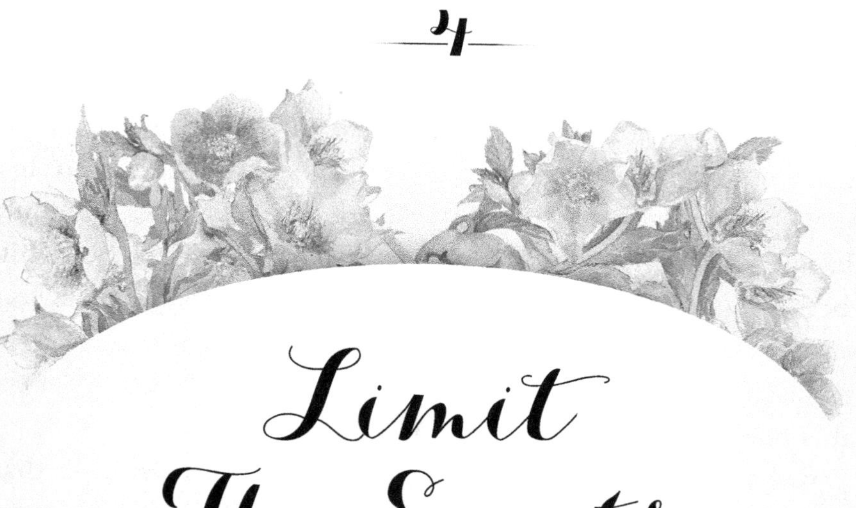

Limit The Sweets

My son, eat honey because it is good, and the honeycomb which is sweet to your taste (Proverbs 24:13).

There is a lot of confusion about sweeteners these days, both artificial and natural. Americans are eating on average 150 pounds of sugar a year.[26] High fructose corn syrups and salad dressings account for a lot of that excess. A steak and two vegetable sides usually have less fat and sugar than a salad with salad dressing when eating out. And it's hard to resist a sweet dessert as the final entrée of a good dinner.

Solomon reminds us that we can have too much of a good thing: "Have you found honey? Eat only as much as you need, lest you be filled with it and vomit" (Proverbs 25:16). To control body weight, most of us must be in tune with our hunger. Eat until you are satisfied, not until you are full (Proverbs 13:25).

Speaking of Honey

Have you ever tasted honey off the honeycomb? That is true sweetness. Try it. My grandpa raised bees. I remember him "suiting up" in a hazmat-type suit with a hooded top. He put on thick gloves, went into his back yard, and lifted the lid off a wooden four-foot-high box while the bees buzzed all around him. Reaching down, he bravely pulled out a honeycomb, dripping with honey still warm from the sun. Then he let us taste the sweet, warm honey, and sometimes he let us eat the comb. I have never tasted anything sweeter on my tongue.

David says, "How sweet are Your words to my taste, sweeter than honey to my mouth!" (Psalm 119:103). Sharing God's words and praying with others will lift their spirits and strengthen their souls.

Bread and Carbs

Carbohydrates are the primary fuel for our brains and bodies. When you talk about carbohydrates, you are talking about the sugar we burn as fuel. The American Diabetes Association at www.diabetes.org has great information regarding sugars and carbohydrates, as well as the National Institute of Health (https://www.nia.nih.gov/health/important-nutrients-know-proteins-carbohydrates-and-fats).

1. Natural simple carbohydrates are the simple sugars found in fruits, milk, and starchy vegetables. Table sugar, sucrose, is considered a simple carbohydrate as well as other natural sweeteners and honey.
2. Processed, "packaged" simple carbohydrates in snack foods such as cake, cookies, candy, syrups, and soft drinks provide a quick energy source but lack all the nutrients and fiber.
3. Complex carbohydrates include nuts, peas, beans, whole grains, fruits, and vegetables. The current recommendations are to eat

more complex carbohydrates because they are chock full of nutrients, natural sugar, and fiber that make you feel full.

Carbs often have a bad reputation when it comes to weight loss. But don't be a Carb-o-Phobic. When choosing a diet, be wary of plans that eliminate an entire food group such as carbohydrates. Instead ask, how many carbs do I need to eat to be healthy?

Both simple and complex carbohydrates break down into the simple sugars that we need for energy. People who promote eating a well-balanced diet often say: "Eat more whole grains" because whole grain breads have more grains and fiber and are less processed and therefore more nutritious. Just remember a portion of carbohydrates is the size of your fist. When you hear a nutritionist say, "Eat more whole grains" this means "choose" more whole grain sources, not double or quadruple the portion.

Exodus 29:2, 23–24, describes a wave offering, which includes a description of bread made from wheat flour. I saw a salesperson at a grocery store promoting "Exodus 29 Bread." The name probably brings up certain images in the minds of people who are familiar with the Bible that somehow make the bread sound better. But don't be swayed by the name of a product. Read labels for nutritional content.

My nutritionist friend said, "Carbohydrates are the primary fuel for the brain and the central nervous system just like God's word is the primary source of fuel for our soul."

The Living Bread

Do you remember when the children of Israel were wandering in the desert? They did not have enough food and water, so God provided them with manna, bread from heaven, to sustain them during their sojourn.

During Jesus' ministry, after the miraculous feeding of the five thousand with the five loaves of bread and two fish and then walking on the sea, some people got into boats and went to Capernaum, seeking Him.

> And when they found Him on the other side of the sea, they said to Him, "Rabbi, when did you come here?" Jesus answered them and said, "Most assuredly, I say to you, you seek Me, not because you saw the signs, but because you ate of the loaves and were filled. Do not labor for the food which perishes, but for the food which endures to everlasting life, which the Son of Man will give you" (John 6:25–27).

Still not understanding, they asked for a sign so they could believe. Jesus answered:

> Our fathers ate the manna in the desert; as it is written, "He gave them bread from heaven to eat." . . . Most assuredly, I say to you, Moses did not give you the bread from heaven, but My Father gives you the true bread from heaven. For the bread of God is He who comes down from heaven and gives life to the world (John 6:31–33).

In that same setting, Jesus said to them, "I am the bread of life. He who comes to Me shall never hunger, and he who believes in Me shall never thirst" (John 6:35). Again, He said, "I am the living bread which came down from heaven. If anyone eats of this bread, he will live forever; and the bread that I shall give is My flesh, which I shall give for the life of the world" (John 6:51).

The children of Israel could not live in the desert without the physical bread sent to them from heaven. Neither can we live without spiritual bread from heaven. Jesus is complete spiritual nutrition, the only true whole grain living bread that we will ever need. Our spiritual health is dependent upon Him. When making healthy spiritual choices in life, we must carefully read the label and look for Jesus as the main ingredient.

Diabetes

A final caution about sugar and carbohydrates. Diabetes is a complicated condition, but whether a person has type 1 diabetes, often called juvenile diabetes (insulin dependent), or type 2 (adult onset) diabetes, a diabetic is unable to break down and utilize sugars adequately. The remaining high circulating blood sugars tend to "sticky up" blood cells and make the person susceptible to clogged arteries which then can lead to a plethora of sight, kidney, heart, circulation, and many other health concerns.

Imagine adding Karo syrup to water. What happens to the consistency of the water? It thickens and moves more sluggishly. This is a simplistic picture of what is believed to happen when too much sugar remains in the blood. Your arteries can be affected. Have you ever had a large sweet snack that puts you in a sugar coma-like state? You may feel like you need a nap and have fuzzy thinking. Good blood sugar control is important.

For diabetics, properly checking and regulating blood sugars will sometimes require a minimum of four finger pricks a day. In addition, the regulation sometimes calls for needle sticks with insulin injections. Diabetics often tell me they feel like a human pincushion.

Although type 1 diabetics are unable to produce insulin that breaks down sugar into a usable form of energy and must be given insulin to live, the rest of us do not have that excuse. Too many sugary treats and indulgences in the food choices we make can make us fat and tired.

Being fat and tired can then lead to spiritual obesity and cause us to become sluggish in our service to God and our fellowman. The church needs alert soldiers for Christ to fend off the devil's wiles, not tired, sleepy, fuzzy-thinking soldiers.

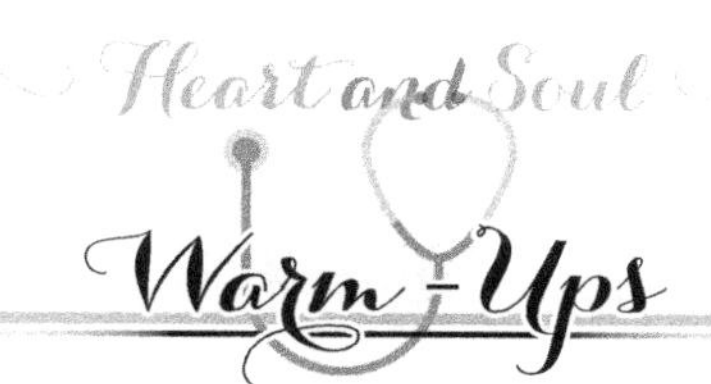

Warm-Ups

- Make a list of some sweet thing you can do for someone instead of giving a basket of cookies or a loaf of banana bread, and then activate your list.
- Discuss why it may be important to eat a protein-filled breakfast. How does protein at breakfast affect your blood sugar? How can you reduce food cravings?
- Set a goal for one week to track calories. Use a tool such as MyFitnessPal to help you be accountable about what you really are eating.
- Think of inexpensive rewards that do not involve food, and treat yourself when you meet a goal.

Soul Stretches

- Paul had a "thorn" in his flesh that he prayed about and dealt with. The Lord declined to remove it. Paul kept his "eye on the ball" anyway and was able to say at the end of his life, "I have fought the good fight, I have finished the race, I have kept the faith" (2 Timothy 4:7–8).

  Runners who keep looking back will not win a race. We can learn a great deal from Paul's attitude. Are you struggling with diabetes, dialysis, cancer, chronic lung disease, or some other "thorn" in the flesh? Pray to God to help you and do everything in your power to control the symptoms. Then decide whether you will allow the disease to rule your life.

- I know many who rise above their infirmities and use their down time to encourage others. They write notes or send texts of encouragement to those around them. Some widows make it a point to take visitors out to eat. One in particular told me, "It is something I can do." Write a list of things you can do for others.
- For those of us not struggling with a thorn in the flesh, let us never forget those around us who are struggling. Send them a text, a note, or bring them a little treat, or call them on the phone. The little things are big to someone.

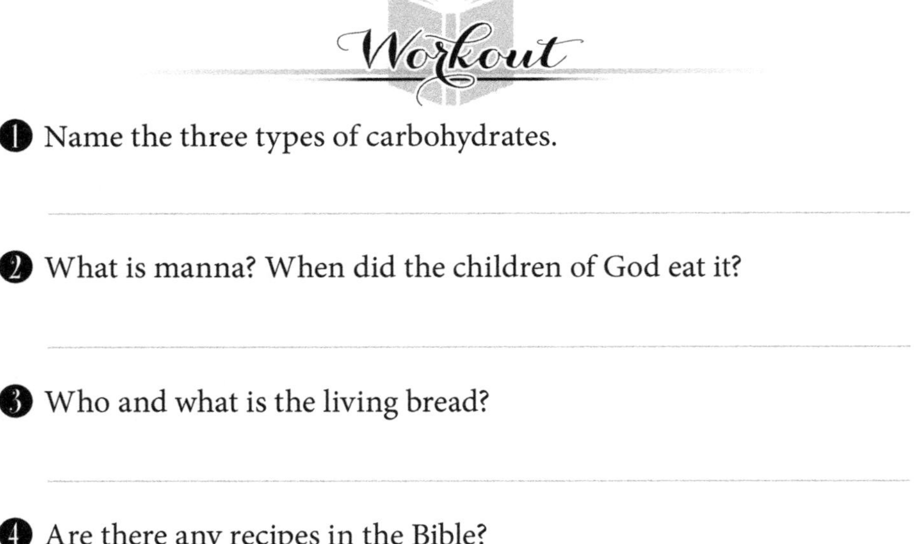

1. Name the three types of carbohydrates.

2. What is manna? When did the children of God eat it?

3. Who and what is the living bread?

4. Are there any recipes in the Bible?

5. When is sugar helpful? Why can sugars be harmful?

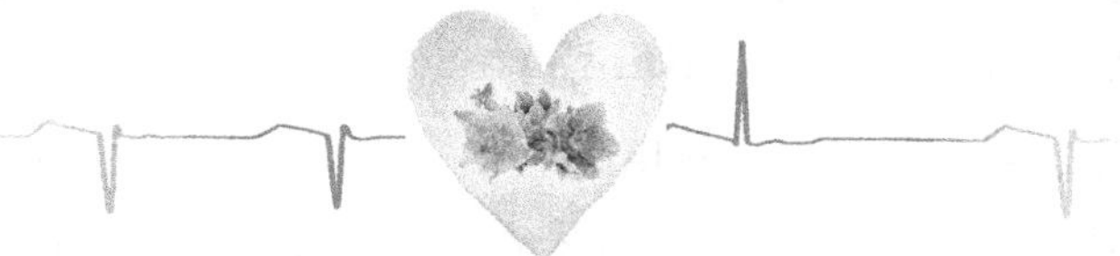

—5—

Activate Daily Exercise

Let us run with endurance the race that is set before us (Hebrews 12:1).

Before we proceed with this chapter, let me remind you that physician supervision is strongly suggested before beginning or changing any exercise, nutrition, or medicinal program. Underlying medical reasons for weight gain, such as thyroid, depression, diabetes, and heart failure need to be ruled out or addressed. Physician input and clearance are especially important if you have co-existing medical problems or symptoms such as chest pain, shortness of breath, or fatigue.

Enjoy Exercise Benefits

The Center for Disease Control generally recommends at least 150 minutes a week, or 30 minutes a day, of aerobic exercise. Unless restricted,

walking is a great example of an aerobic large-muscle, weight-bearing exercise. You should be able to "talk" but not "sing" throughout the exercise. Here are some other benefits of physical exercise:

- Exercise can control your weight; raise your HDL, the healthy part of your cholesterol panel; and lower your triglycerides. This one-two punch, according to the Mayo Clinic, is enough to reduce, or even prevent, the development of cardiovascular disease and stroke.[27]
- Exercise aids in the prevention or management of high blood pressure, type 2 diabetes, stroke, depression, arthritis, falls, and even certain types of cancer.
- Exercise raises the "feel good" endorphin hormones released in your brain.
- Exercise can improve how you feel about your appearance, thus boosting confidence.
- Exercise is known to boost energy and improve sex life and even promote sleep.
- Exercise can just be a great release and fun.
- Many insurance plans also cover a consult with a nutritionist who may help you develop a plan of attack or offer you discounts and credits for the exercise and wellness programs you attend. What a wonderful benefit!

Core Exercises

In addition to strength exercises, core exercises need to be an important part of your routine.[28] Shaping up the muscles around your trunk and pelvis are key to a strong back, hips, and abdomen, not to mention better balance and stability. The "muffin top" in women (that fatty roll

overhang above the waistband that appears when we slide our jeans up) and the "spare tire" belly fat, often associated with middle-aged men, are more than unattractive and uncomfortable. They are limiting.

- The extra fat and weight cause us to move off center and shift our center of balance enough to contribute to falls.
- It can prevent us from bending over to cut our toenails or tie our shoes.
- That fat around our core can cause us to injure our back because of the shift in our balance.
- It can contribute to knee, foot, hip, and back problems.

Have you ever heard that old song with the line, "The head bone is connected to the neck bone"? When one part of our body is out of place, it affects many other parts. Our spinal column is made up of donut-like discs that stack from our tailbone to our neck. When out of alignment, the likelihood of pain and limiting muscle spasms is increased.

Adults lose muscle as they age and become weaker. Strength training does have benefits. Lifting weights boosts metabolism, reduces osteoporosis, and builds muscle. This can be done at home or in a gym.

Deciding not to live with these mostly self-imposed and preventable problems is the first step to overcoming them. But knowing what to do and doing it are two very different things. The adage, "You can lead a horse to water but you can't make him drink," is so true. We have to decide in our minds and hearts that we are going to get in shape physically and spiritually before we will succeed. If we think we can, then we will. Our service to the Lord is dependent upon our ability and willingness to work. Make this decision now: "Today is the day I will get rid of my physical and spiritual limitations and barriers." Only you have the power to do this.

There's an App for That

If you are a smartphone user, there are many free applications to assist you with your weight loss and fitness programs.

- *MyFitnessPal*, a free application, allows you to track your food, exercise, and water, and then break down your calories into fats, carbs, and proteins. You can also set a weight goal and track your progress.
- *Restaurant Nutrition* is another free app that allows you to make smarter choices by planning ahead when you are eating out.
- *NIH BMI calculator* is yet another free tool from the National Institute of Health that will assist you in finding out what your healthy weight range should be.
- *ChooseMyPlate.gov* is a free app put out by the USDA and has valuable visuals and resources for understanding portion control and food choices.

For those who are 50 pounds or more overweight, a "weight loss" or bariatric physician may be the most appropriate person to assist you in helping manage your weight loss.

Exercise Selflessness

Our spiritual body also needs some strength and core training. When it comes to our spiritual body, we should exercise selflessness, which can be just as painful and difficult as bodily exercise. Sometimes it hurts while we are going through it, but we reap the benefits of being in shape.

We live in a me-centered world. Paul reminds us: "Let nothing be done through selfish ambition or conceit, but in lowliness of mind let each esteem others better than himself" (Philippians 2:3). When we

take the time to do something for someone else, we are often the one who gets the most out of it. It can be a small thing such as holding a door for a mother and her baby or an elderly person with a cane. Calling someone on the phone or texting is cheap and fast.

"Let each esteem others better than himself." In our days of rush and hurry, we often forget that the most important and meaningful thing we can give to our children or neighbors or friends is our time. Time is opportunity. Put first things first.

Paul said, "But I discipline my body and bring it into subjection, lest, when I have preached to others, I myself should become disqualified" (1 Corinthians 9:27). Get fit spiritually. Paul speaks of running a good race and disciplining his body athletically to parallel what preparation and discipline we need to make to run our Christian race and engage in battle with Satan.

"But reject profane and old wives' fables, and exercise yourself toward godliness" (1 Timothy 4:7). Verse 8 says, "For bodily exercise profits a little, but godliness is profitable for all things, having promise of the life that is and of that which is to come."

When we prioritize our time, it is clear that growth in godliness is more beneficial than exercising to become fit. We have the Great Physician to help guide us with our spiritual exercise and growth. When we are sick, we want a physician who is a healer and a comforter. Jesus is that Physician.

Picking up those around us when they are down is sure to build spiritual muscle. Paul reminds us, "Bear one another's burdens, and so fulfill the law of Christ" (Galatians 6:2). So don't forget to lift weights. You don't have to do it alone. Share the load.

Lessons from Geese[29]

Milton Olson

Fact 1: As each goose flaps its wings it creates uplift for the birds that follow. By flying in a V formation, each goose increases its flying range by 71 percent, as compared to its distance when flying alone.

Lesson—People who share a common direction and sense of community can get where they are going quicker and easier because they are traveling on the thrust of one another.

Fact 2: When a goose falls out of formation, it feels a sudden drag and a loss of lift because of the increased air resistance. The loner moves quickly back into formation to take advantage of those benefits provided by the bird immediately in front of it.

Lesson—If we have as much sense as a goose, we stay in formation with those headed in the direction we want to go. We are willing to accept their help and give our help to others.

Fact 3: When the lead goose tires, it rotates back into the formation and a fresh goose flies to the point position.

Lesson—It pays to take turns with hard tasks and leadership. As with geese, people are interdependent on each other's skills, capabilities, and unique arrangements of gifts, talents, or resources.

Fact 4: The geese, flying in formation, honk to encourage those leading the flock to maintain their speed.

Lesson—We need to make sure our honking is encouraging. Group encouragement increases production. The power of encouragement—to stand by one's heart or core values and encourage the heart and core of others—is the quality of honking we seek.

Fact 5: When a goose gets sick, wounded, or shot down, two geese drop out of formation and follow it down to help and protect it. Then they launch out with another formation or catch up with the flock.

Lesson—If we have as much sense as geese, we will stand by each other in difficult times as well as when we are strong.

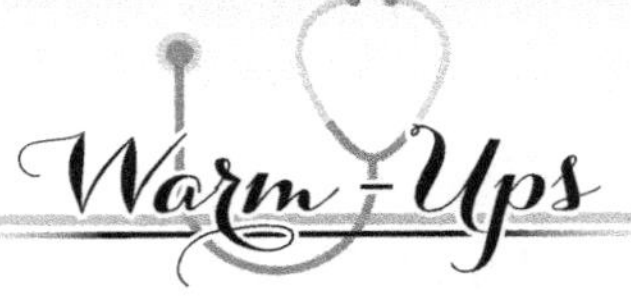

- Find the free MyFitnessPal app. Plug in your favorite foods and look up nutritional content and macros pie chart. Try the app for one week. Do the same with Choosemyplate.gov and evaluate your portion choices.
- Evaluate in minutes-a-week, how many exercise minutes you accomplished this past week. Note: Activity is not the same as exercise. Exercise raises your heart rate for a period of time and sustains it. Is there room for improvement?
- Discuss the difference between activity and exercise.

Soul Stretches

- Read 1 Timothy 4:7–8. How is Paul commanding us to be godly? Perform a soul checkup on your daily activity toward godliness. What exercises and activities can you do to become spiritually athletic?
- Meditate on the idea that bodily exercise may enhance your spiritual life and put your positive thoughts into action.

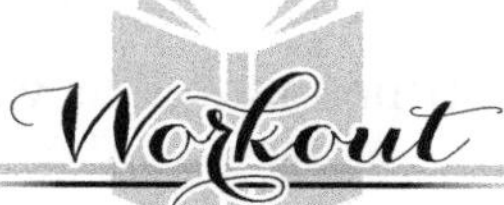

Workout

1. How can you exercise and practice selflessness?

2. Why is exercise important for the church?

3. List some ways to build spiritual muscles. (See Galatians 6:3.)

4. What kind of goose are you? A flapper, a honker, a leader? Discuss.

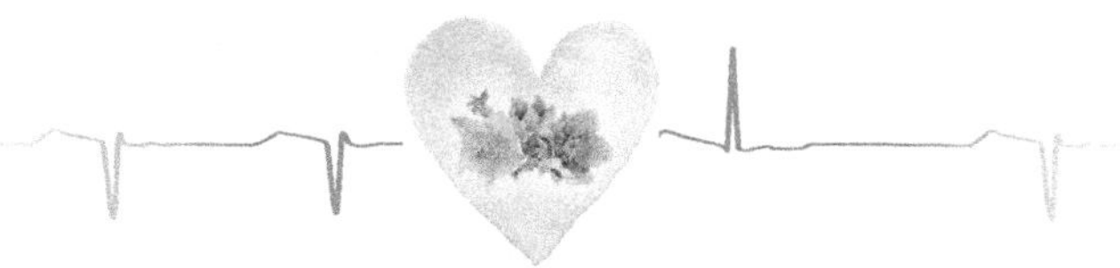

—6—

Exercise The Senses

Oh, taste and see that the Lord is good; blessed is the man who trusts in Him! (Psalm 34:8).

What are you chewing on? What you choose to put into your mouth and your mind matters. We've talked about the significance of what goes into your mouth. The same is true for the mind. And what goes into one affects the other.

Webster defines *food* as "materials used by the body to sustain growth, repair, and to furnish energy." Your body takes what you put into your mouth and breaks it down into tiny particles. These tiny particles are then carried by the blood through the blood vessels to every cell in the body to be used immediately, to be stored for later use, or to be eliminated.

Your spiritual heart, the intellect, also receives what you put into it and breaks it down to use or store. What are you tucking away on a

daily basis in the recesses of your mind? It is foolish to think what you watch on TV or see at the movies or hear in the words of songs will not affect you. Children repeat what they hear, sometimes when they hear it only once. And adults remember more than they like to think. How many times do the lines from a movie or lyrics of a song come to mind even years after you have heard them?

The Senses

The decisions you make about what you choose to eat are personal and often driven by your moods and emotions. Multiple body systems and all five senses—sight, smell, hearing, taste, and touch—are involved in the simple act of eating

What do you think of when you smell an apple pie baking? Mom? Maybe you remember how it felt when you helped her pick and peel the apples. Maybe you helped to cut them up and roll out the dough with a rolling pin. The smell of apples baking in the oven brings back memories of home and family.

At a family get together, you may have been served a big breakfast with fried apples, eggs, sausage links, bacon, and homemade biscuits. The sound of sausage and bacon frying and the smell of coffee brewing and biscuits baking awakens even the usual late sleepers. How does that make you feel?

Maybe you grew up baking homemade chocolate chip cookies after the Friday night game. The smell of the cookies and the taste of the chocolate bring back warm feelings of celebration.

Feelings of pure pleasure can be linked to a person's favorite foods. Think about what happens when you see or smell something yummy. Your body starts responding. Your mouth begins to salivate long before you put in the first bite. Once you savor it with your tongue, chew it, and swallow it, your heart is triggered to send extra blood to the

stomach to break down that food into tiny parts for use or storage or elimination.

Morgan, my little West Highland terrier, loved Thanksgiving turkey, and we gave her some as a treat every year. She licked her chops and smacked her lips when we even said the word *turkey.* Her ears perked up in anticipation of just a little bite of turkey, no matter what month of the year.

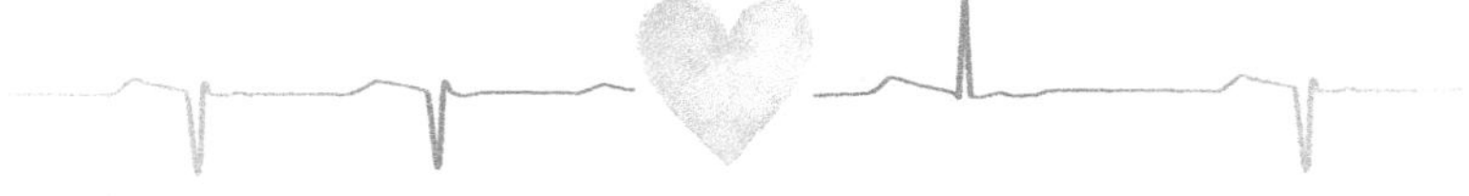

"For the ear tests words
as the palate tastes food" (Job 34:3).

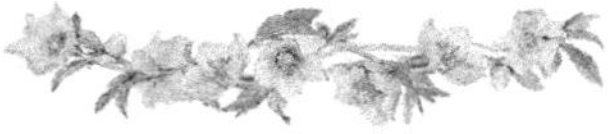

God gave you uniquely placed taste buds on your tongue to discern what tastes good and what tastes bad. Some people like sour things and others do not. Pizza is one of those foods that can make people feel good because they often have it with family and friends or at a party or some other fun event. It is warm and cheesy and gooey. The point is, you choose what to put into your mouth.

There is nothing wrong with taking pleasure in eating. When my granddaughter Haley was one year old, she really liked to eat and often touched her food while she was eating it. Food can be a comfort. My mom brewed black tea and made toast when I was sick. Perhaps your mother fixed hot chicken noodle soup when you were sick with a cold, and now a whiff of that steaming liquid brings you feelings of comfort.

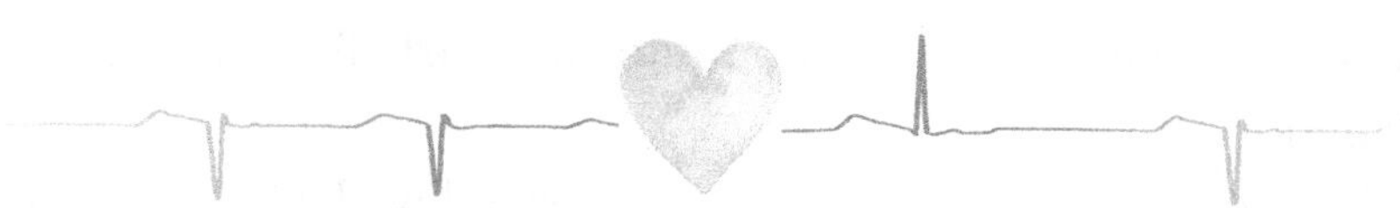

"Your words were found, and I ate them, and Your word was to me the joy and rejoicing of my heart; for I am called by Your name, O Lord God of hosts" (Jeremiah 15:16).

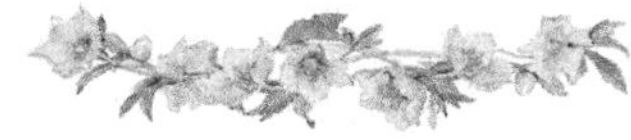

Digesting the Word

Every day you get up and decide what you are going to put into your mouth—and your mind. Perhaps one of your friends opens her eyes and reaches for her Bible, while another feels for her cell phone or the remote to click on the morning news. What about you?

Jeremiah was a major prophet of God. His name means, "Whom God has appointed." According to Jeremiah 15:16, when he digested the Word of God, he understood joy and rejoicing. The Word of God was a pleasure to him.

A Taste of Trust

David tells us that if we seek the Lord we shall not lack anything. True comfort and nourishment will come only through God. He will take care of us. "The Lord will not allow the righteous soul to famish, but He casts away the desire of the wicked" (Proverbs 10:3). We will never starve if we obey. That is a promise. God will take care of us.

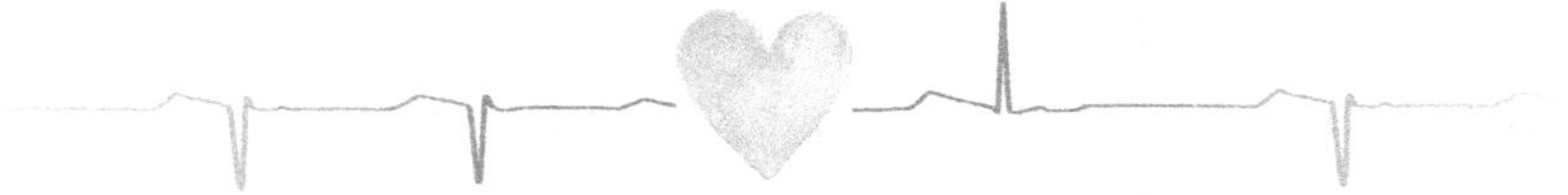

"Oh, taste and see that the Lord is good; blessed is the man who trusts in Him! Oh, fear the Lord, you His saints! There is no want to those who fear Him. The young lions lack and suffer hunger; but those who seek the Lord shall not lack any good thing" (Psalm 34:8–10).

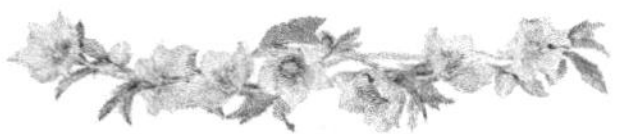

Very often, though, God's care is not in the ways we anticipate. So Solomon encourages us,

> Trust in the Lord with all your heart,
> And lean not on your own understanding;
> In all your ways acknowledge Him,
> And He shall direct your paths.
> —Proverbs 3:5–6

The idea that the Lord will direct my very path is reassuring. But I have a responsibility there also. I must look to God and accept that direction and trust Him no matter where that may lead.

Before we moved to North Carolina back in the 1980s, we were down to our last paycheck, and I was nine months pregnant. Then we responded to a telephone solicitation and allowed a Kirby vacuum cleaner salesman to demonstrate his product by cleaning our carpet. The manager himself came to do the job. He obviously noticed that I was near to giving birth, so he listened as we explained why we could not make a purchase that day. Next thing we knew, my husband, Terry, got his first computer programming job for the Kirby Company.

Trust, according to *Strong's Enhanced Dictionary,* means to be confident, to be sure. The word *heart (kardia)* means the center, your will

and intellect, that part of you that decides what to do.[30] *Direct* means to make your path straight.[31] How comforting it is to know that God will direct your path, if you will trust Him. It just may not be in the way you expected.

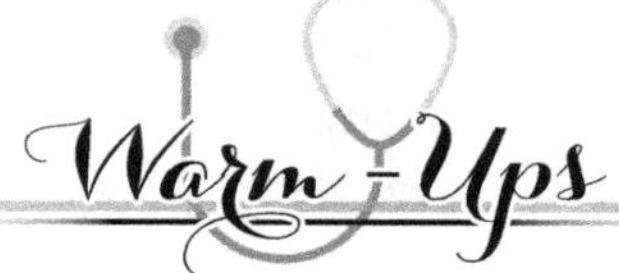

Warm-Ups

- Look up the word *satiety.* How can we achieve satiety with food?
- Pass out a small snack to the group. Which of our five senses are used when we eat? Discuss appetite, hunger, and satiety.

Soul Stretches

- Discuss Proverbs 13:25.
- Make a list of questionable subjects or language that would affect you spiritually. Place the list close by when you watch TV and keep track of how many times in a week you were exposed to those things on your list. At the end of the week you may have a tough decision to make about your TV viewing habits. Memorize Philippians 4:8 to motivate you in your decision.

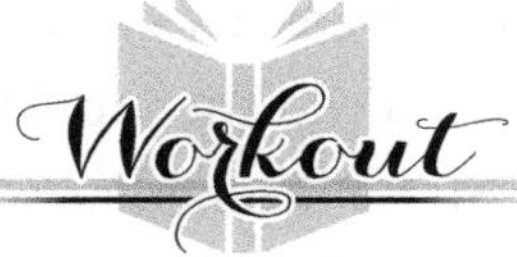

Workout

❶ How important are the five senses to our eating?

2. Why do we label certain foods "comfort foods"? What are yours and why?

---

3. Do you have any "comfort verses" you go to in times of stress?

---

4. Read Hebrews 5:14 from several translations. How does training your spiritual senses relate to maturity? Give an example of how a new Christian might have trouble discerning good and evil.

---

5. What kinds of feelings did Jeremiah have after digesting the Word? Did it bring comfort to him?

---

6. Discuss the meaning of Psalm 34:8–10.

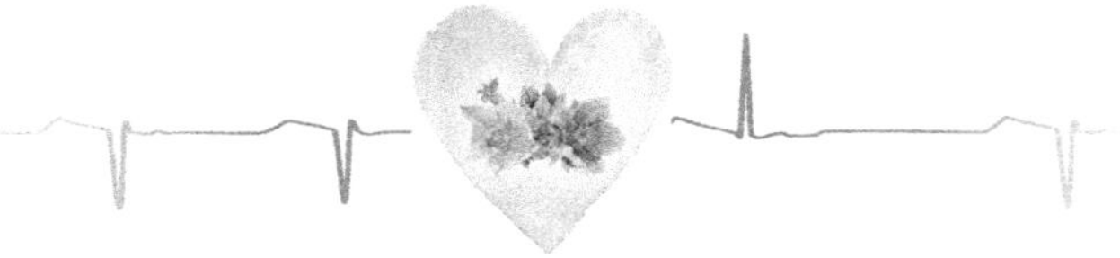

—7—

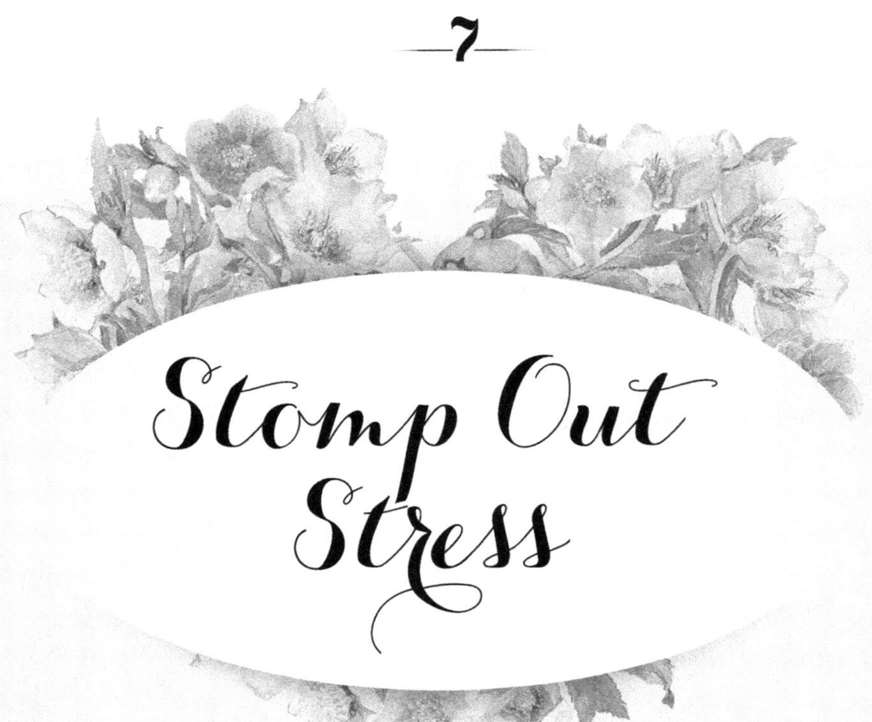

Stomp Out Stress

Do not worry about tomorrow, for tomorrow will worry about its own things. Sufficient for the day is its own trouble (Matthew 6:34).

Stress has real physical consequences. When your body is stressed, it responds as if it were under attack. It activates your "fight or flight" hormones—epinephrine and norepinephrine—and can:

- increase your heart rate.
- increase your blood pressure.
- cause your liver to produce more cholesterol.
- cause your pituitary gland to throw out more cortisol and sugar.[32]
- decrease your immune system and make you more susceptible to disease.

Managing stress is critical. If you are a diabetic, you know your blood sugar runs higher whenever you are sick, overly stressed, or recovering from surgery. Asthma, Crohn's disease, and even certain cancers are linked to chronic unmanaged stress. In the Sermon on the Mount, Jesus reminds us that our heavenly Father already knows what we need and encourages us not to worry. Life is more than food and clothing. In Matthew 6:33 He admonishes followers to put first things first, saying, "Seek first the kingdom of God . . . and all of those other things shall be added to you."

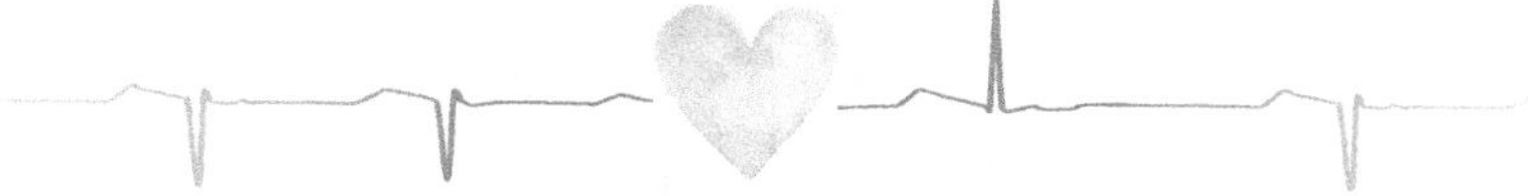

"Do not worry about your life, what you will eat or what you will drink; nor about your body, what you will put on. Is not life more than food and the body more than clothing?" (Matthew 6:25).

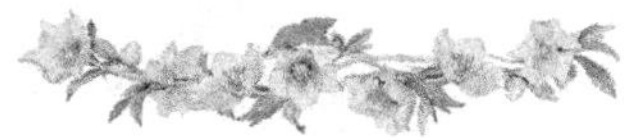

A Stressful Encounter

Elijah's encounter with Queen Jezebel is a perfect example of what happens when we allow stress to become uncontrolled and take over our lives.

In 1 Kings 18–19, we learn that King Ahab and Queen Jezebel were worshiping idols instead of God; they trusted the prophets of Baal. Elijah, which means "God is YHWH," was a prophet of God.[33] To prove to the people there is only one God, he challenged the prophets of Baal to an altar-burning contest. The prophets of Baal were unable to convince their god to light the fire on the altar despite leaping, calling out to him, and even cutting themselves. Elijah egged them on, saying, "Either [your god] is meditating, or he is busy, or he is on a journey, or perhaps he is sleeping and must be awakened." Of course, Baal did not light the altar.

Then Elijah gathered all the people together and poured four pots of water on the altar—not once, not twice, but three times! There was so much water it filled a trench around the altar. Elijah said, "Lord God of Abraham, Isaac, and Israel, let it be known this day that You are God in Israel and I am Your servant, and that I have done all these things at Your word." God sent down fire that consumed not only the wood, stones, and dust, but also the water in the trench. After this, Elijah said, "Seize the prophets of Baal." He was then able to execute all of them.

When King Ahab told Queen Jezebel what had happened, Jezebel sent a messenger to Elijah saying, "So let the gods do to me, and more also, if I do not make your life as the life of one of [the prophets of Baal] by tomorrow about this time." In other words, by this time tomorrow Elijah's life would be over.

When Elijah learned of Jezebel's plan, he left immediately and traveled south about a day's journey. He stopped to rest under a broom tree and prayed to God that he might die. Elijah slept until an angel awakened him, fed him a cake, and gave him water. But Elijah lay back down, so God sent the angel a second time who again awakened him and said, "Arise and eat, because the journey is too great for you." He arose and ate. That food sustained him for forty days and forty nights as he traveled to Mount Horeb and took refuge in a cave, where he was visited by the Lord.

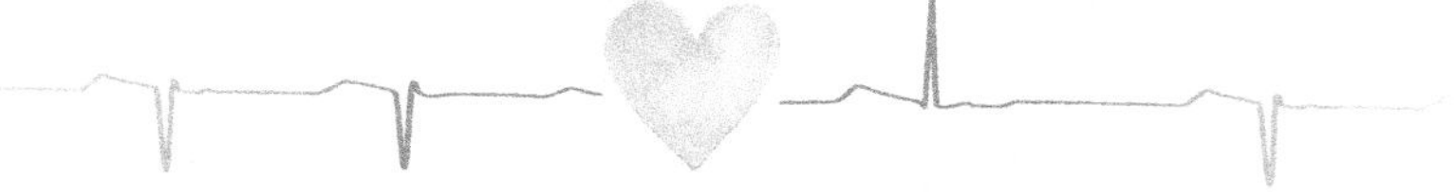

"For if anyone is a hearer of the word and not a doer, he is like a man observing his natural face in a mirror; for he observes himself, goes away, and immediately forgets what kind of man he was" (James 1:23–24).

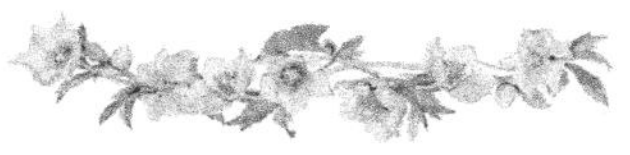

Stress Can Lead to Depression

Stress per *Meriam Webster* is a state of mental tension and worry about perceived problems in your life, job, etc. Stress can sometimes drive people into a depressed state. Elijah was highly stressed and fearful for his life. He isolated himself, stopped eating, wanted to sleep all the time, and prayed to God that he would die. Dr. Jerry Martin, dean of the School of Human Services at Amridge University and licensed counselor, stated at the 2012 Polishing the Pulpit weekend, "Elijah did have all the signs of a clinically depressed person."

A person dealing with depression can be difficult to be around. Here are some things to look for:

- She isolates herself and often wonders why no one has missed her.
- She seems to play hide-and-seek with brothers and sisters in the church.
- Sometimes you misinterpret her absence and speculate incorrectly about why she isn't present.
- She refuses to answer the phone for an extended period of time.
- When you go to visit, you find all the shades pulled down.
- If you could go inside her home, you would probably find no groceries—not even junk food.
- A passing glimpse of her would reveal an unkempt, perhaps ghostly figure.
- She may be in a hospital—or worse—may be contemplating suicide. Look and listen to see if she has thought through a plan with details about how and when or that she has started giving away her favorite things. This is a truly serious matter. Seek professional assistance immediately and do not leave her alone.

You may truly be tempted to run away from such a person, especially if you think she is just feeling sorry for herself. However, your reluctance to become involved is not in her best interest.

God did not leave Elijah (cf. 1 Kings 19:14–16). He gave him a job—to go and anoint a new king. So Elijah anointed Jehu and threw his mantel on a new prophet, Elisha. In so doing, he commissioned Elisha to take his place. Maybe a lesson can be learned from this story about how to handle in a godlier manner those who are dealing with depression.

God recognized Elijah's needs and miraculously intervened by using an angel to provide him with food. The Bible doesn't say how God performed that miracle or what was in that food, but it's clear that it was sufficient to comfort and sustain Elijah when he needed it.

Maybe you should follow this example and strive to recognize those struggling with depression:

- Nourish and nudge them without losing patience.
- Help them get back to God's work instead of waiting for disaster to strike.
- Help them seek needed professional attention, whether by counseling or medicines that are necessary to sustain them.
- Remember not to leave them alone.

You Are Not Alone

The last thing God did for Elijah was to reassure him by telling him that he was not alone in his rejection of Baal, as he thought. There were seven thousand others like him (1 Kings 19:18). It is important to know that Elijah was emotionally on top of a mountain before he fell into the valley of depression. He won a great victory over King Ahab and Queen Jezebel and the prophets of Baal, only to plunge into intense fear under Jezebel's threat to take his life. If you pray with those

who are in a depressed state and let them know that God is with them, that can be as comforting and healing as any medicine. Don't underestimate the healing power of your presence, prayer, and concern for the welfare of a fellow Christian.

The Thanksgiving and Christmas holiday seasons are very hard for many people. These are times filled with the laughter of children, dear family members, and friends. However, for those people who have suffered loss during these times, the holidays are especially painful. Holiday seasons provide an opportunity to comfort others who are beset with sadness. Remember to look around and reach out to those who have holes in their hearts and shine your Christian light to lead them out of the paralyzing depths of depression.

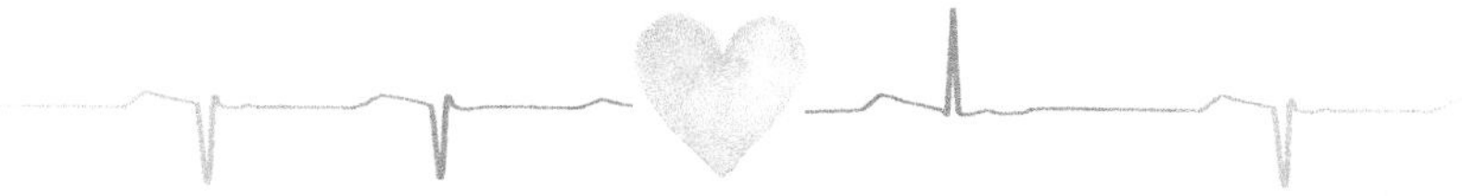

"Two are better than one, because they have a good reward for their labor. For if they fall, one will lift up his companion. But woe to him who is alone when he falls, for he has no one to help him up. Again, if two lie down together, they will keep warm; but how can one be warm alone? Though one may be overpowered by another, two can withstand him. And a threefold cord is not quickly broken" (Ecclesiastes 4:9–12).

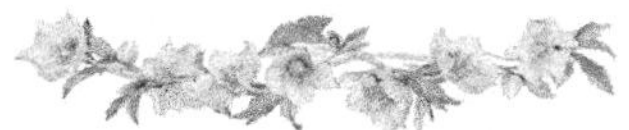

Develop Healthy, Godly Friendships

Close intimate relationships are heart healthy. One of the best ways to manage stress is to confide in a good friend. You need to develop strong intimate relationships with God and your brothers and sisters in Christ.

- Proverbs 27:17: "As iron sharpens iron, so a man sharpens the countenance of his friend."
- Proverbs 17:17: "A friend loves at all times, and a brother is born for adversity."
- Proverbs 18:24: "A man who has friends must himself be friendly, but there is a friend who sticks closer than a brother."
- Proverbs 12:26: "The righteous should choose his friends carefully, for the way of the wicked leads them astray."

That last passage is a reminder that you must be careful about your choice of friends because of their influence on you.

Cultivate godly friendships by nourishing each other, nudging each other, as did the angel with Elijah, more than once if necessary. When you look back at the bad times in your life, you might be surprised to notice who stood with you. Did they give you the solution you needed, or did they just listen while you did the problem-solving on your own?

My best friends ever are those who have led me into a circle of Christians who helped me to find comfort in times of trouble. They spent more time listening than they spent offering a solution. I do believe that is why God gave us one mouth and two ears. We can listen to others in stereo, and comprehend their needs before we open our mouths in response.

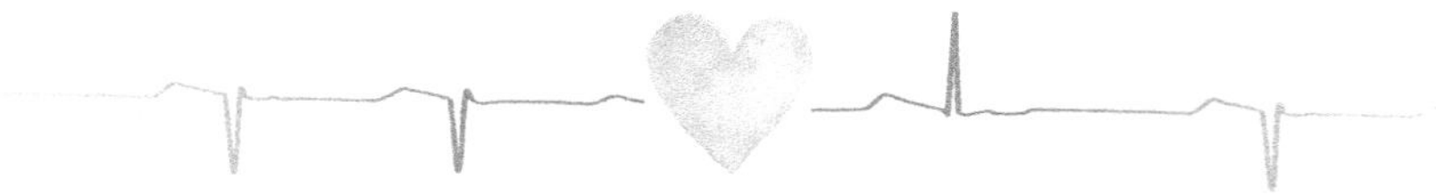

"Confess your trespasses to one another, and pray for one another, that you may be healed. The effective, fervent prayer of a righteous man avails much" (James 5:16).

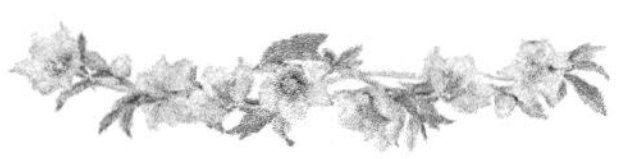

Remember to Pray

Scripture tells us that God answers prayers and keeps promises.

> Confess your trespasses to one another, and pray for one another, that you may be healed. The effective, fervent prayer of a righteous man avails much (James 5:16).

> Now to Him who is able to do exceedingly abundantly above all that we ask or think, according to the power that works in us, to Him be the glory in the church by Christ Jesus to all generations, forever and ever. Amen (Ephesians 3:20).

I don't know about you, but if I have an abundance of something, then I have more than I need. This passage says God can do more than you can ask or think. That is an amazing concept since most of us can ask for a lot.

The point is to ask for help from God and then believe that He can help you. Matthew tells about a man who came to Jesus telling how His disciples could not cure his epileptic son. Jesus asked that the son be brought to Him for healing. His disciples came to Him privately and asked why they were unable to help the boy. Jesus said to them,

> Because of your unbelief; for assuredly, I say to you, if you have faith as a mustard seed, you will say to this mountain, "Move from here to there," and it will move; and nothing will be impossible for you (Matthew 17:20).

It is most reassuring that God is there and hears and answers our prayers if we believe—even if our faith is as small as a pinhead. Later Jesus said,

> Assuredly, I say to you, if you have faith and do not doubt, you will not only do what was done to the fig tree, but also if you say to this mountain, "Be removed and be cast into the sea," it will be done.

And whatever you ask in prayer, believing, you will receive (Matthew 21:21–22).

Food Is Not the Answer

Many people dealing with emotional issues, such as stress and depression, look for comfort in food. They feel that something is missing, like there is a hole in their heart, and they try to fill it with food. My patients have told me they binge eat the most when they are feeling nervous, stressed, depressed, lonely, grieving, or ashamed, or guilty about something. They mistake their true emotion with hunger and often overeat or binge eat.

Binge eating occurs when a person eats anything accessible in large amounts quickly, and often when they are alone. They frequently eat alone because they are ashamed of the amount of food they are eating and want to do it secretly, which usually adds to their guilt and depression. They get caught in a circle of binge eating, guilt, and depression.[34]

Depression and emotional eating are serious matters. If you are experiencing these issues, seek medical help immediately. Food is not the answer. Fill that hole in your heart with God and spiritual things. We just cannot do it alone. In Philippians 4, Paul reminds us to meditate on things that are true, noble, just, pure, lovely, virtuous, and of good report (v. 8). Later in the chapter he reassures us, "I can do all things through Christ who strengthens me" (v. 13). In other words, when we feel our weakest, Christ will strengthen us if we ask in prayer and seek out Christian friends to help us. We must become new women. It does take setting our minds on things above, not on things of the world (Colossians 3:2).

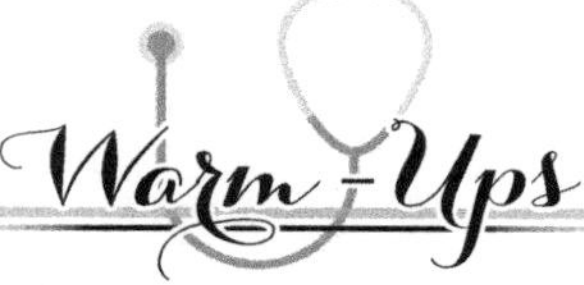

Warm-Ups

- Discuss the psychological component of emotional, binge, or compulsive eating.
- Do an inventory of your relationships in life and then think about what you liked to do together. Is there an association with food?
- If some of the driving forces of an eating disorder are abandonment, rejection, and inability to self-nurture, what can be done?
- I was told the following by a "card carrying" emotional eater, that focusing on God and others has changed her. She told me she has learned that life has become bigger than food, now that she is a Christian. She said she has learned now to fill the empty spot in her heart with God. What a blessing and encouragement she is. God bless her open heart. What can you learn from her experiences?

1. Emotional/compulsive and binge eaters can have triggers. Each person has her own trigger whether it is loneliness, depression, guilt, or lack of self-worth. It is eating or not eating for any reason other than hunger.
2. Binge eating food is like an allergy of the mind. Those suffering from this eating disorder have a complex relationship with food. They eat so as not to feel an uncomfortable emotion. They substitute food for an emotional need.
3. Learn to be "present and conscious," and become a "mindful" eater.
4. To overeaters, food becomes their constant and always gives them the feeling they want, but then afterwards the guilt sinks in.

5. A binge eater will isolate herself, eat quickly, or buy bags of cookies or chips and hide them from her spouse to prevent feeling judged.
6. Membership in a support group may not cure a person, but it will raise awareness.

Soul Stretches

Close your eyes and think about the most peaceful place you have ever experienced. Then read Philippians 4:7. The peace of God "surpasses" all our understanding. From previous verses in Philippians 4, write yourself a recipe for that peace.

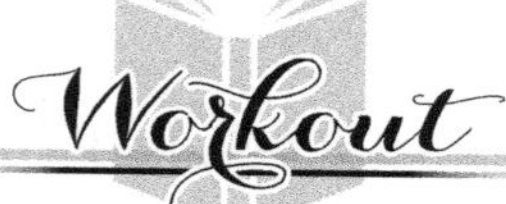

Workout

❶ What are the consequences of excessive worry?

❷ What are the consequences of depression spiritually?

❸ Meditate on Philippians 4:6–7; 1 Peter 5:6–7; and Matthew 6:34. Consider the seriousness of worry. Why shouldn't these commands be respected as much as "love one another"? Why are these commands about worry and anxiety ignored?

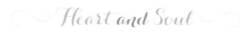

4. According to Proverbs 17:17; 18:24; James 5:16; and Ecclesiastes 4:9–12, what are the characteristics and value of a friend?

5. Read 1 Peter 5:6–7 and Ecclesiastes 4:9–12. What is the danger of isolating ourselves?

6. How does a man "sharpen" the countenance of his friend? Read Proverbs 27:17.

7. Ecclesiastes 4:9–12 says two friends are better than one, but a three-fold cord is not quickly broken? Why is this?

8. Matthew 17:20 talks about belief and a mustard seed. How are believing friends who pray and fast for you in times of trouble beneficial?

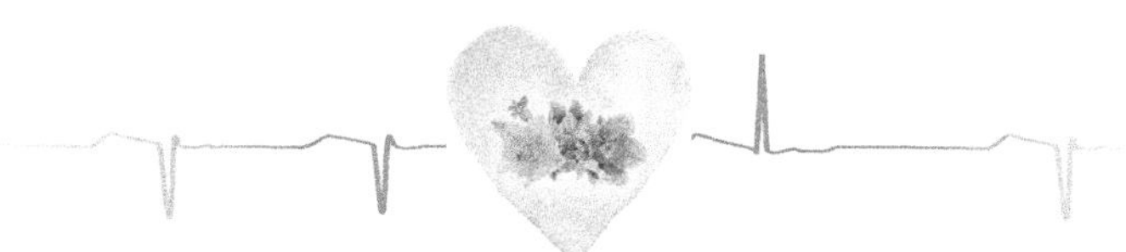

8

Douse Anger Flames

He who is slow to anger *is* better than the mighty, and he who rules his spirit than he who takes a city (Proverbs 16:32).

Do you remember seeing the old cartoons on Saturday morning of an angry man turning red and smoke or steam coming out of his ears? That picture was often accompanied by a loud screaming train whistle. Have you ever become so angry that you imagined smoke coming out of your ears? Probably you would have heard someone say, "Calm down!"

More than likely we all have been around an impatient, frustrated, exasperated family member or some other distressed person, as they reach for a cigarette for tranquility. They may look at you and say, "After all, it's legal and what's the harm? It keeps me from blowing my top."

Here's the danger: the chemicals in tobacco set you up for narrowed, clogged arteries that accelerate your risk for heart attack or stroke. Cigarette smoking is the "single most preventable cause of death in the U.S."[35]

A heart needs plenty of oxygenated blood from the lungs and needs to be well fed with nutrients carried in the blood through the blood vessels to do the amount of work it does every day. The average heart is just the size of your fist. Every single minute of every single day we draw a breath it pumps blood 60–100 times through blood vessels that, if laid end to end, would circle the earth twice.

Although the hazards of the chemicals and toxins in cigarettes and the damage to the blood vessels, lungs, and heart are widely publicized, people still smoke. Why? Is it a habit? My patients tell me they cannot quit because they are addicted. They have made smoking a habit that is usually associated with some activity, such as drinking a cup of coffee in their favorite chair after breakfast, or driving their car when they are stressed.

One of my patients, a mortician, said that when he receives bodies that have been autopsied, he knows immediately which ones have been smokers because of the gray film lining around all the organs. "It resembles the gray shiny, filmy, residue found on the bottom of an ashtray," he said. So stop smoking; put out the flames!

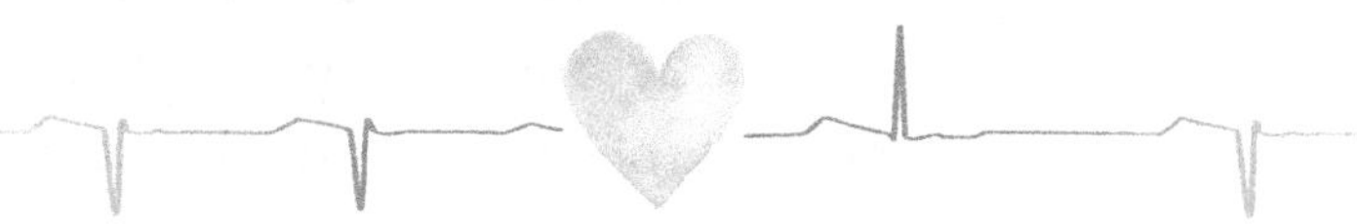

"Cease from anger, and forsake wrath; do not fret—it only causes harm" (Psalm 37:8).

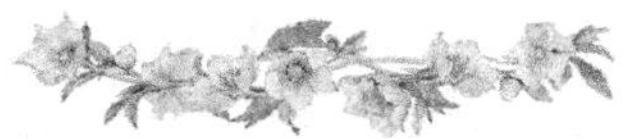

A Ticking Bomb

I used to watch my mother can green beans using a pressure cooker. After cooking for the needed time, the pressure valve began to jiggle and then hiss rhythmically with a tsh-tsh-tsh sound. When the pressure got too high inside, the top would pop up, make a screaming sound, and reduce pressure as steam rushed out and immediately transformed itself into a cloud of hot vapor. I have come to believe that if we do not experience an emotional release on occasion, something inside us "pops."

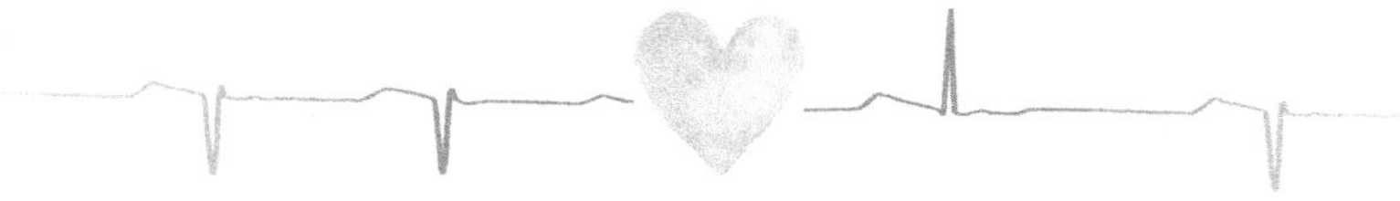

"But now you yourselves are to put off all these: anger, wrath, malice, blasphemy, filthy language out of your mouth" (Colossians 3:8).

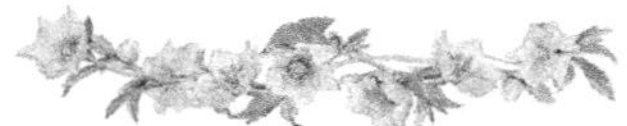

Anger and hostility can cause pressure to build up inside of you. In the heart world, medical professionals used to worry about the type A personality, the gung-ho person who runs circles around her co-workers. She is the one who gives a hundred percent of herself a hundred percent of the time.

Today, however, we know that the person most at risk for heart disease is the angry/hostile type.

- She keeps everything bottled up, harboring ill feelings, hostility, and anger.
- Her emotions seem to sit in her chest, simmering and smoking, steaming and ticking like a time bomb, until one day they explode.

- She often has time-urgency issues and trouble waiting and may be tapping her watch or tapping her foot in a nervous tic-like manner.
- She may become irate and impatient on the highway and turn into a road-rage driver, honking, swearing, or waving a gun.

Let It Go!

If you are hanging on to disappointments of the past or stewing over obstacles of the present, allowing them to simmer deep inside your chest without ever dealing with the true issue, you are creating a very unhealthy atmosphere for your heart. Are you making a habit of nursing a grudge? Anger and hostility can cost you not only your relationships but also your life. Find a way to build a bridge. If you are hanging on to the past, you will never be able to move forward. Look for ways to work through it and vent constructively. You can never lead others to Christ if you are "smoking." Figure out what the problem truly is and then come up with a plan. Often the problem comes to light when you write it down.

Paul offered both admonitions and solutions to the Ephesians:

> Let all bitterness, wrath, anger, clamor, and evil speaking be put away from you, with all malice. And be kind to one another, tenderhearted, forgiving one another, even as God in Christ forgave you (Ephesians 4:31–32).

It is hard for people to hate us when we are kind to them despite their shortcomings.

Self-Control

Having an outlet for anger has many health benefits. For example, taking a brisk walk may avert disaster. Exercise actually raises the endorphin level. Endorphins are the feel-good hormones. If we are abrupt with those around us, fling our arms, or stomp our feet, it can appear

as if we are angry even when we are not. The same is true at church services. Rushing past those around us or pushing past people to "save our seat" can present us in a negative light.

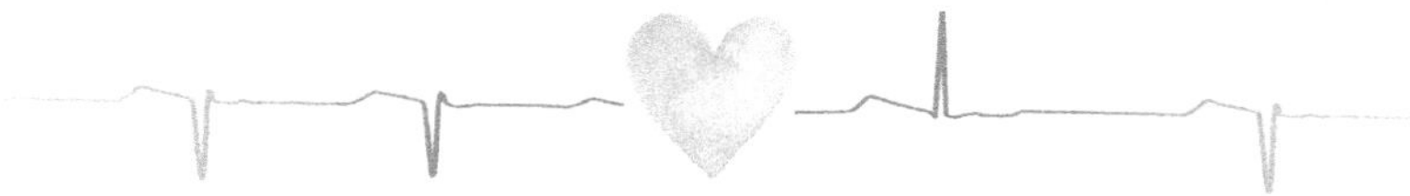

"He who is slow to anger is better than the mighty, and he who rules his spirit than he who takes a city" (Proverbs 16:32).

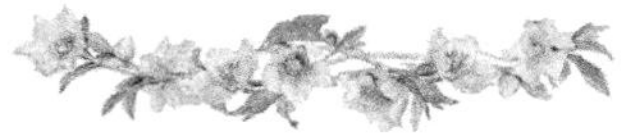

People who don't "fly off the handle" quickly are better than warriors capable of taking over a whole city. The person who can properly deal with her emotions shows incredible self-control and strength. If you are married to an individual with this character trait as I am, you are fortunate indeed.

Solomon also said, "A soft answer turns away wrath, but a harsh word stirs up anger" (Proverbs 15:1). A tender or soft or delicate response can stop an argument before it begins. The word *harsh* can mean painful, grievous. I have sat in meetings that have become volatile in reaction to the tone of the speaker's voice. The manner in which we speak is very important. Oral communication skills should be a part of our school curriculum, because so many misunderstandings occur when the speaker unintentionally uses poor techniques.

Some people seem to be looking for a fight. "A wrathful man stirs up strife, but he who is slow to anger allays contention" (Proverbs 15:18). In other words, a furious man can cause a quarrel, but a man who is able to control his anger can defuse a volatile situation and bring about peace. Jesus says, "Blessed are the peacemakers" (Matthew 5:9). We must exercise self-control in regard to anger and hostility, if

we ever expect to win others to Christ. The lyrics of "Angry Words," written by Horatio R. Palmer in 1867, are timeless. These words apply today as much as they did two-and-a-half centuries ago when they were written.

> Angry words. O let them never,
> From the tongue unbridled slip,
> May the heart's best impulse ever,
> Check them ere they soil the lip.
>
> *Refrain*
> Love one another, thus saith the Savior,
> Children obey the Father's blest command,
> Love one another, thus saith the Savior
> 'Tis the Father's blest command.
>
> Love is much too pure and holy,
> Friendship is too sacred far,
> For a moment's reckless folly,
> Thus to desolate and mar.
>
> Angry words are lightly spoken,
> Bitt'rest thoughts are rashly stirred,
> Brightest links of life are broken,
> By a single angry word.

In a New York minute, you can see good relationships break and close friendships dissolve. That can happen when someone loses his cool and spouts off angrily. Be the peacemaker that Jesus called "blessed" in the Sermon on the Mount. It takes two to argue, so resolve not to argue. Be like the character John Wayne portrayed in the

1952 movie *The Quiet Man* who refused to be forced into a fight. Once you lose your cool, you will lose your influence to lead others to Christ.

Jonathan

In 1 Samuel 18:6–11, we read how the women took to the streets singing the praises of David after he killed Goliath. From that day forward, Saul became jealous and obsessed with killing David, so much so that he threw a spear at him. Jonathan discovered Saul's true feelings and warned David (1 Samuel 19). Later Saul and Jonathan argued about David, so Jonathan knew Saul was determined to kill him.

> So Jonathan arose from the table in fierce anger, and ate no food the second day of the month, for he was grieved for David, because his father had treated him shamefully (1 Samuel 20:34).

Notice that Jonathan developed a "fierce anger." The more I study about Jonathan, the more I have learned to respect and admire his character. He did everything he could to right a wrong, and used his anger to take constructive action to protect David.

Jonah

Jonah, on the other hand, allowed his anger to take control of him and drive him to disobey God. In Jonah 1:1–17, God told Jonah to go to Nineveh and warn them that God knew about their wickedness. Instead, Jonah paid a fare and got on a boat to run from his responsibility and from God. So the Lord sent out a great wind on the sea to the point that the ship was going to be broken apart. When the mariners found out their troubles with the boistrous waves were due to Jonah's flight from God, they became afraid and asked Jonah to talk to God and make the sea calm. Jonah finally told them to throw him overboard.

The Lord had prepared a great fish to swallow Jonah, and he was in its belly three days and three nights. When Jonah repented of his

actions, the Lord spoke to the fish, and it vomited Jonah onto dry land (Jonah 2:10).

For the second time, God told Jonah to go to Nineveh and preach the message that in 40 days Nineveh would be overthrown (Jonah 3:4). We are told the people from the least to the greatest, including the king, believed God, fasted, put on sackcloth, and repented, so God spared them.

Jonah, however, became so displeased and angry that he prayed that God would take his life. Although he acknowledged that God was gracious, merciful, slow to anger, and abundant in loving kindness, he allowed his own anger to dictate his behavior and disobey God. He went to the east side of Nineveh and made himself a shelter to sit in the shade and see what would happen to the city. God prepared a plant to provide shade and then used the plant to teach Jonah about compassion for others. God reminded him that there were more than 120,000 innocents in the city of Nineveh that needed his assistance (Jonah 4:1–11). Jonah had allowed his emotions to dictate his actions rather than do the Lord's will. His anger was misplaced.

Balaam

In Numbers 22 we read the story of Balak and Balaam. Balak of Moab sent his servants to pay Balaam the soothsayer to curse the people of Israel (vv. 5–6). God became angry with Balaam for going with Balak's men (v. 22). When Balaam rode on his donkey to meet with Balak, God sent an Angel with a sword to stop him. Now the donkey saw the Angel and turned the other way, but Balaam, not seeing the Angel, struck the donkey to turn her back on the road.

The donkey protected Balaam two more times from being killed by the sword of the Angel of God. Then God opened the mouth of the donkey, and she said to Balaam, "What have I done to you, that you have struck me these three times?" (v. 28).

After this, God opened Balaam's eyes, and he saw the Angel of the Lord standing in the way with His drawn sword in His hand. And Balaam said to the Angel of the Lord, "I have sinned, for I did not know You stood in the way against me. Now therefore, if it displeases You, I will turn back" (v. 34).

Then the Angel of the Lord said to Balaam, "Go with the men, but only the word that I speak to you, that you shall speak" (Numbers 22:35).

So Balaam went with the princes of Balak and prophesized four times but did not curse the children of Israel as Balak had hoped.

> Then Balak's anger was aroused against Balaam, and he struck his hands together; and Balak said to Balaam, "I called you to curse my enemies, and look, you have bountifully blessed them these three times!" (Numbers 24:10).

God foiled Balak's evil plan against the children of Israel using Balaam the soothsayer.

Jesus

Finally, let's look at how Jesus handled anger. In Matthew 21, Jesus came upon a disgusting sight of greed at the temple. Jesus came upon people who, no doubt, were out to make a profit from those traveling and unprepared for their sacrifice at the temple. We read,

> Then Jesus went into the temple of God and drove out all those who bought and sold in the temple, and overturned the tables of the money changers and the seats of those who sold doves. And He said to them, "It is written, 'My house shall be called a house of prayer,' but you have made it a 'den of thieves'" (Matthew 21:12–13).

We must stand up for what is right whenever possible, but does this mean we should become angry and hurt those around us to make our point? We must use our influence to help others decide to go in the

direction of God. We cannot make them do it. They alone must choose to put God first in their lives.

We have studied many examples of anger in action. Angry words cannot be taken back. Angry texts, voicemails, and emails live forever. Channeling our anger and taking steps to right wrongs in a constructive manner can show Christ to others. Channeling our anger and blowing off steam by exercising is a great way to cope.

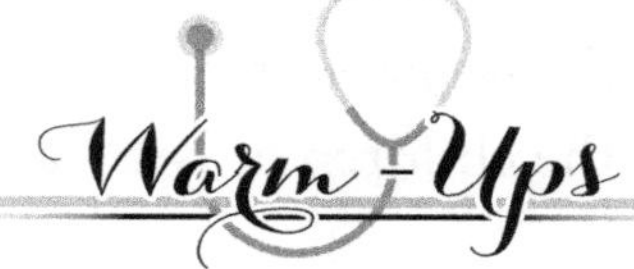

- Anger increases your blood pressure and heart rate and causes a cascade of fight-or-flight hormonal and bodily reactions. For me, one of the easiest ways to burn off anger is to take a brisk walk. Some of you have shared with me that when you are short tempered and angry, you count to 10 before speaking. Share other ways you have been successful in managing your temper and anger.
- Research anger management resources you have in your community or on the job.
- Discuss the hormonal reactions inside your body when you become angry. Do we think rationally when angry? Discuss the anger in road rage.
- Name some synonyms of "anger." Name some antonyms. Then share instances when you saw "red." How can your antonym list help you to keep your cool?

Soul Stretches

How many times have we, like Balaam, become angry, maybe at our spouse or children about something we thought they were doing, only to find out we were completely wrong? Pray now that God will assist us to use our anger constructively and lead others to Christ by our humility and example.

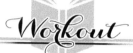

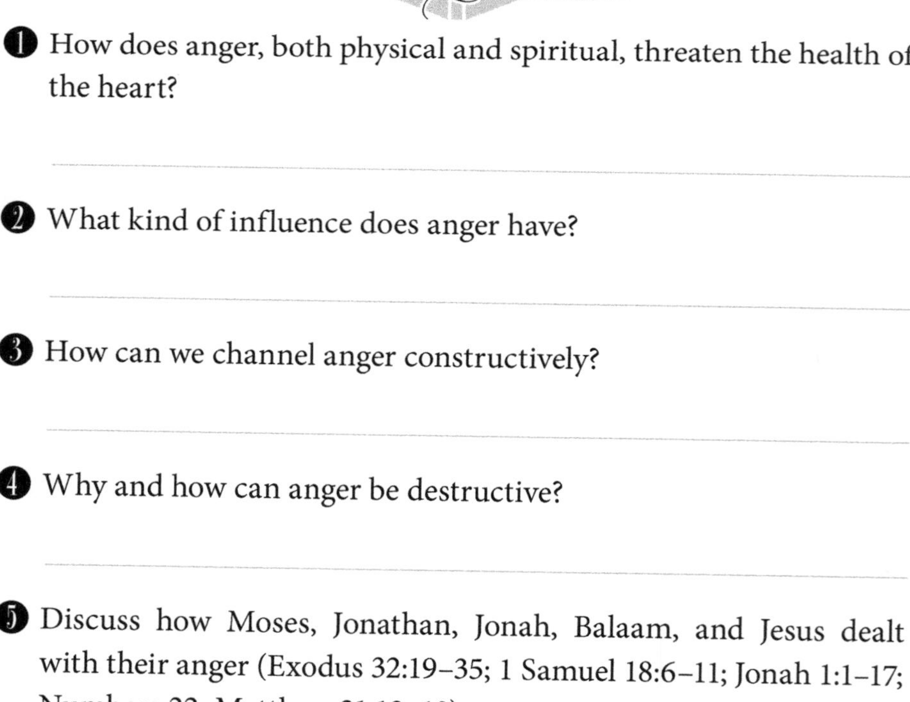

Workout

1. How does anger, both physical and spiritual, threaten the health of the heart?

2. What kind of influence does anger have?

3. How can we channel anger constructively?

4. Why and how can anger be destructive?

5. Discuss how Moses, Jonathan, Jonah, Balaam, and Jesus dealt with their anger (Exodus 32:19–35; 1 Samuel 18:6–11; Jonah 1:1–17; Numbers 22; Matthew 21:12–13).

❻ What steps can we take to avoid losing our cool and influence?

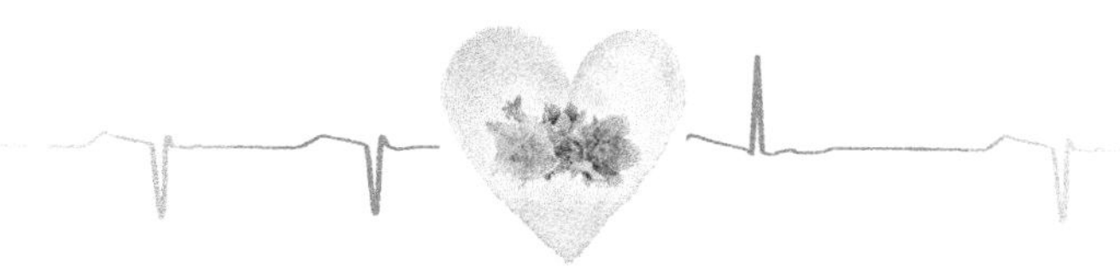

9

Tame The Tongue

Even so the tongue is a little member and boasts great things. See how great a forest fire a little fire kindles (James 3:5).

Words Fitly Spoken

We can motivate and influence others to evaluate their lives and adopt a healthy lifestyle both physically and spiritually with the words we choose. While planning for a ladies' retreat, a dear sweet sister sent me a brief text. It said, "Just thinking about you." What a comfort this was to me. She knew I was preparing to teach while balancing work and family issues, and she recognized the challenges I would be facing that week. Her prayers and kindness helped to carry me through.

My friend knew just what to say and when to say it, but using encouraging words can be tricky. We don't want to offend or make matters

worse, so we often choose to say or do nothing. There are times, however, when someone you know loses a dear family member or loses her job or is having family problems and desperately needs some comforting. What a comfort that little pat on the arm or a hug can be. Technology can never take the place of human love and touch that we need to thrive. Your presence with friends during hard times speaks volumes about how much you care, even if you say nothing at all.

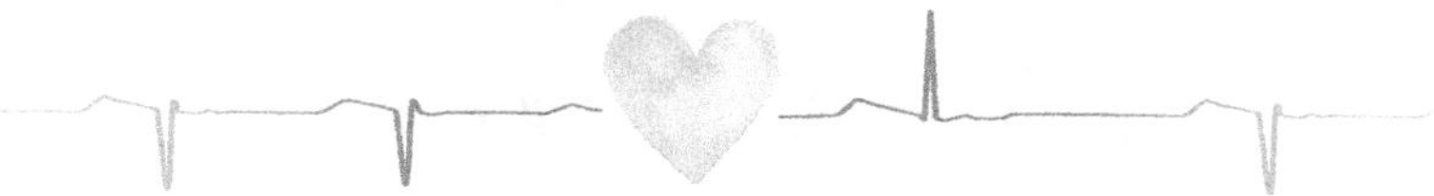

"Even a fool is counted wise when he holds his peace; when he shuts his lips, he is considered perceptive" (Proverbs 17:28).

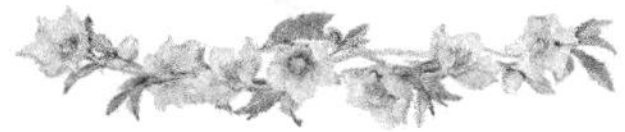

Planting and Harvesting

I grew up in Ohio around cornfields and grape vineyards. That turned out to be a valuable life experience. I learned that the ground must be readied at a certain time of the year in order to plant and grow good crops. Just like there is a right time to plant and harvest, there is a right time to speak and a right time to keep our mouths shut. Wise is the person who understands that.

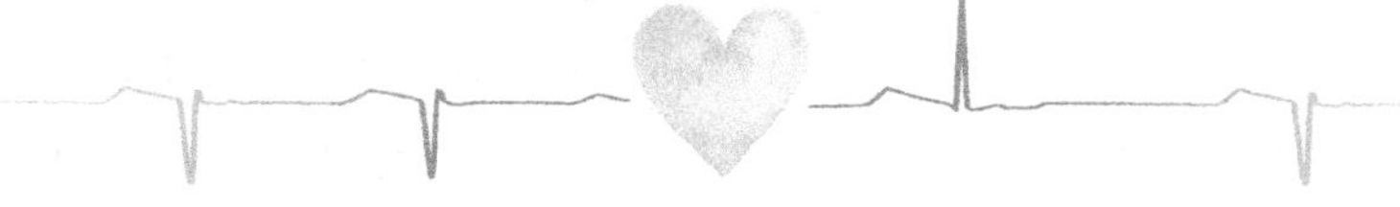

"To everything there is a season, a time for every purpose under heaven . . . a time to plant, and a time to pluck what is planted . . . a time to keep silence, and a time to speak" (Ecclesiastes 3:1–7).

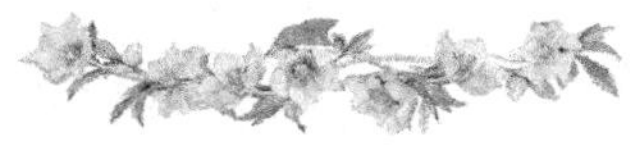

What we put into our mouths is important, but also important is what comes out of our mouths. Our mouths have the ability to send weak members or visitors running out the church door, so be careful with your words. Wise men have often quoted Abraham Lincoln, "It is better to remain silent and be thought a fool, than to open your mouth and remove all doubt" (also attributed to Confucius and Mark Twain).

The Great Boaster

Our true nature is most often revealed by our speech. "The tongue is a little member [of our body] and boasts great things" (James 3:5). The tongue produces great destruction or creates major change, both good and bad. We can both curse and praise with it.

So we can have a better understanding, James, believed to be the brother of Jesus, describes the power of the tongue as:

- A bit in a horse's mouth (James 3:3).
- A rudder (James 3:4).
- A tiny flame (James 3:5).

A Horse's Bit. Having grown up around horses weighing nearly a ton, I am still amazed that the tiny bit we put into their mouths can control their speed and direction.

A Rudder. Have you ever waded in the ocean? Its power is humbling. Even shin high, the waves can knock you down. But a sea captain, using a tiny rudder, can control a giant ocean liner in the face of fierce winds and waves. In a similar way, an uncontrolled tongue can and will wreak havoc.

A Flame. Equally amazing is that a tiny ember left at a campfire can burn great forests, scorching thousands of acres of timberland. What an ugly scar that leaves behind on the mountainside. The nakedness and barrenness are hard to bear.

James finally said, "Who is a wise man and endued with knowledge among you? Let him shew out of good conversation his works with meekness of wisdom" (James 3:13 KJV).

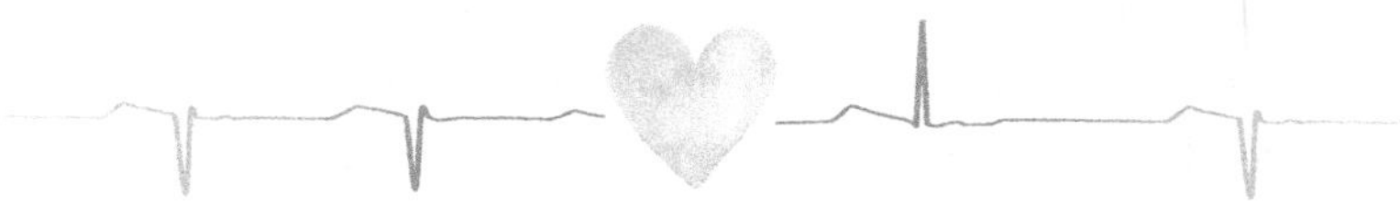

"The discretion of a man makes him slow to anger, and his glory is to overlook a transgression" (Proverbs 19:11).

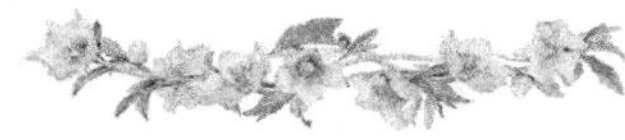

Going Viral

Facebook and other forms of social media have become securely anchored in our lives. We now stay in contact with those around us, even those who live on the other side of the globe. It is great to see pictures of family and friends. However, written communication lives on and has a life all its own. My own words when misunderstood have spun off into the universe and come back in a form I did not recognize. Be careful with words you say and even more careful with words and pictures you might write or post. Parents and many families have been hurt by undisciplined speech online.

Going viral is dangerous and deadly in the medical world. Theories about the way a new strain of Ebola virus spreads have monopolized the news in times past, and we still don't know for sure how it spreads. Contact with a virus by air, body fluids, or touch can infect healthy people, guilty of nothing more than being in close proximity to the "germ."

"Going viral" in the technology and information world is equally damaging. Good people are "infected" by simply having access to the "germs" spread with technology.

Please do not misunderstand. The technology we use can be a great resource for information sharing. It has the potential of reaching those looking for God in remote places. People can now search for the truth from the privacy of their homes. The shut-in can participate in worship remotely. That can be a wonderful thing.

Dirty Laundry in Public

But the Internet is not a place for children. Neither is it a place to air your dirty laundry or anyone else's, unless you are prepared to see it on the front page of a newspaper. Many reputations have been damaged by careless words online. Careless words have always had the potential to hurt; however, with technology, careless words can literally reach the whole world in less than a second. Once the words are out, it is impossible to take them back or control them. Speech can become metastatic.

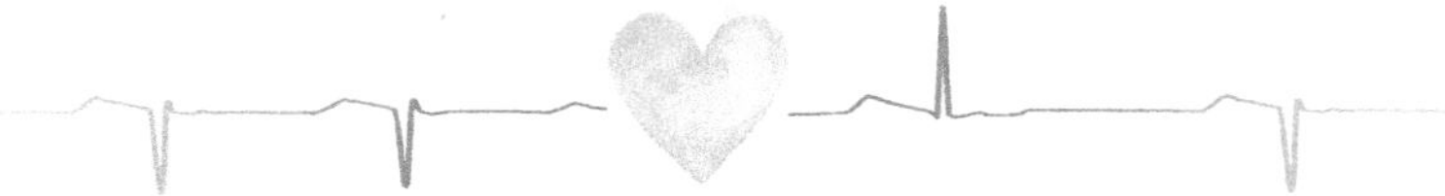

"He who keeps the commandment keeps his soul, but he who is careless of his ways will die" (Proverbs 19:16).

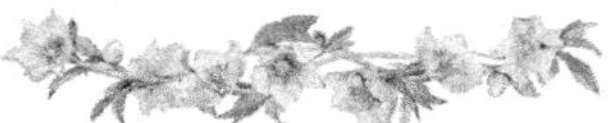

Carelessness in medical practices can lead to death. If health-care providers do not practice proper hand washing, deadly infections can kill the innocent. If we are careless in regards to lifestyle, we can kill others or ourselves prematurely. Think about those practicing illicit sex. Sexually transmitted diseases can lead to sterility and death. Avoid potentially compromising situations and relationships, and save yourself and your loved ones from trouble, complications, and heartache. Learn

to recognize such things and avoid them. Listen to your God-given ability and intuition. Your actions can have lifelong physical and eternal spiritual consequences.

Please be careful with your words. The saying, "Loose lips sink ships" originated during World War II on propaganda posters to advise servicemen to avoid careless talk that might be used against the United States by the enemy.[36] Use your computer wisely. Damaging words posted online have led to suicide. Worse yet, damaging words can cause us to lose our souls and jeopardize the souls of others.

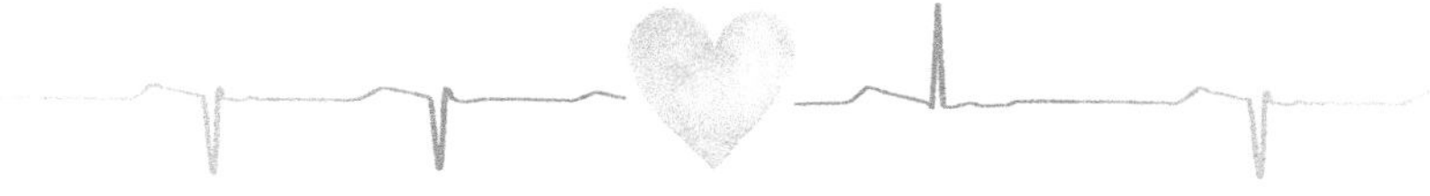

"But I say to you that for every idle word men may speak, they will give account of it in the day of judgment" (Matthew 12:36).

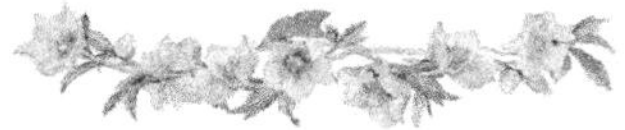

Ambassadors for Christ

We all expect ambassadors at the United Nations to represent the beliefs and cultures of their countries in the way they dress and treat others and the way they speak. We should expect nothing less from Christians who are ambassadors for Christ. Hold the gossip. The contents of our hearts will rise to the surface.

Those people who watch their mouths closely get into less trouble than those who tell all. Your associates are judging you by what comes out of your mouth.

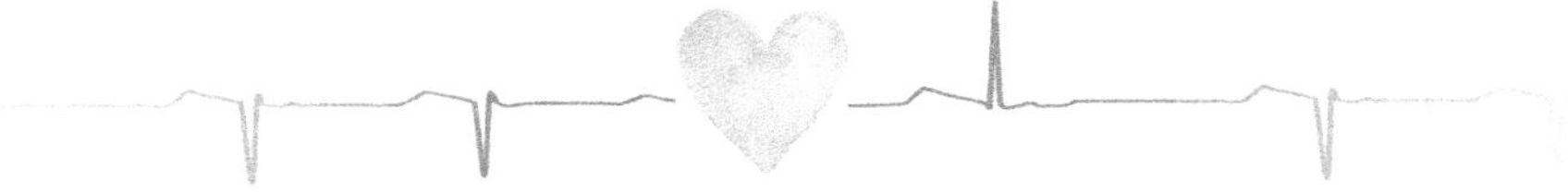

"Keep your heart with all diligence, for out of it springs the issues of life. Put away from you a deceitful mouth, and put perverse lips far from you" (Proverbs 4:23–24).

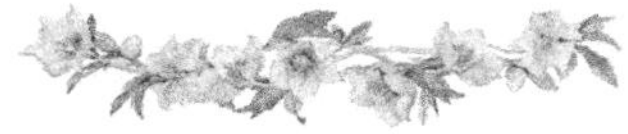

A Lying Tongue

Have you ever watched a spider weave its web? It crisscrosses back and forth and all around until it makes a beautifully intricate and patterned web. That web is coated with a sticky substance, perfect for capturing prey. Liars also weave intricate stories, but instead of catching their prey, they are caught in their own webs.

Think about Ananias and Sapphira. In Acts 5:1–11 they tried to deceive Peter and the apostles into believing they were more generous than they really were, giving all they had from the sale of their possessions. In Acts 5:4 Peter told them, "You have not lied to men but to God." Their lie cost them their lives.

Scam artists beware.

> Whoever causes the upright to go astray in an evil way, he himself will fall into his own pit (Proverbs 28:10).

> Bread gained by deceit is sweet to a man, but afterward his mouth will be filled with gravel (Proverbs 20:17).

If you have been a deceiver, your deeds will come back to haunt you. The thrill of having pulled a quick one on someone may feel sweet at first, but Solomon says afterward, your "mouth will be filled with gravel." Although I do not make a habit of eating gravel, I have tasted

a few as a child when I fell off my bike. They are nasty and gritty, and the taste did not leave my mouth very quickly. Again, Barney Fife's famous line comes to mind; it is "ill-gotten gain." God sees your actions and every secret thing.

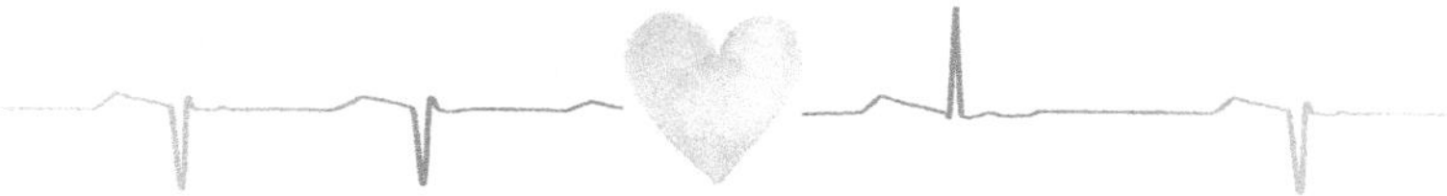

"The words of a talebearer are like tasty trifles, and they go down into the inmost body" (Proverbs 18:8).

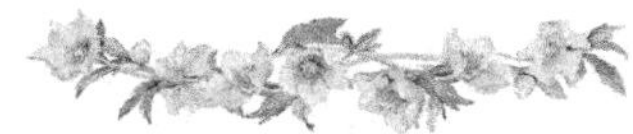

The Taste of Gossip

Gossip is like a tasty trifle. A talebearer makes the story being told so appealing that you cannot wait to hear the end. *Tasty* is defined as being "appealing, interesting, and palatable." The word *trifle* is defined as a "dessert." In other words, a tasty trifle is something sweet you want to savor and taste.

Have you been a victim of gossip? It is hard to change the perception of people, even if the tale is completely false. Lives can be ruined and relationships lost. Jesus reminds us: "Out of the abundance of the heart the mouth speaks" (Matthew 12:34). We associate a nuclear waste byproduct dump as toxic, and nobody wants one in their backyard. In the '70s people even carried signs that said, NIMBY (Not in My Back Yard). Likewise, nobody wants to be associated with toxic gossip.

Remember, gossip is a toxic cancer—metastatic, in fact. It spreads like wildfire and when we make the decision to do the spreading, we must remember that life and death are in the power of our tongue. It takes two to gossip. If you find yourself in a situation where gossip is occurring, walk away. Go to the object of the gossip and stop the

cancerous spread. As was said earlier in this chapter, our actions can have lifelong physical and eternal spiritual consequences.

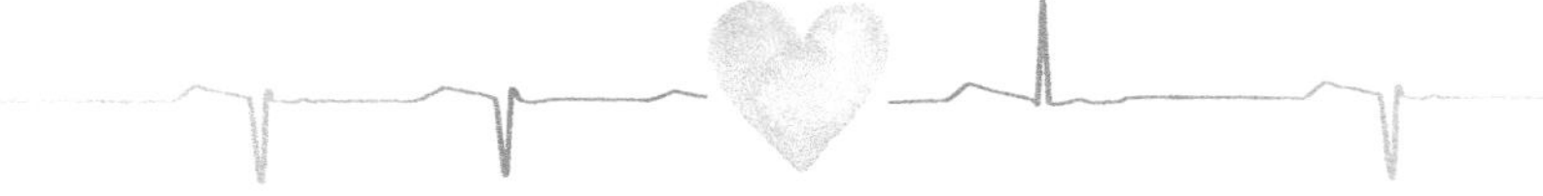

"Death and life are in the power of the tongue, and those who love it will eat its fruit" (Proverbs 18:21).

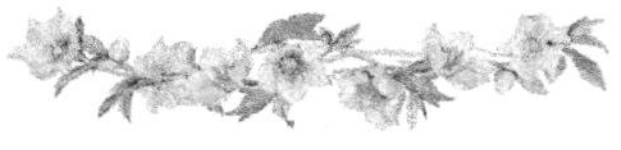

Warm-Ups

Play "Telephone." Before class, write a sentence on a piece of paper. Have the person next to you read it and then whisper the sentence to the person next to her. Without passing the paper, have each person repeat the message to the person next to her. At the end, have the last person write down what she was told and read it out loud. Compare it to what was written initially.

Soul Stretches

Some lies are considered harmless by the world. We even call them *white lies* or *fibs* to make them sound better. This week make yourself a "liar's bank" out of an unused butter bowl or cottage cheese container—something you can't see through. Then every time you catch yourself telling a "white lie," drop a quarter into the bank. At the end of the week, count how many quarters you have. Be prepared to discuss

this with the class next week, maybe even sharing one or two that you told.

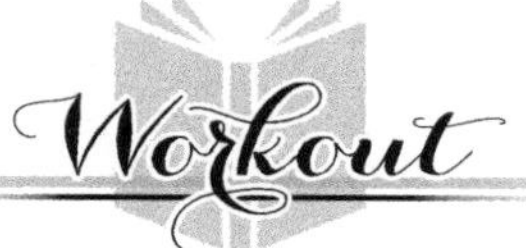

Workout

1. Read Ecclesiastes 3:7. Discuss a time we should be silent.

2. Read James 3:1–10 and discuss suggestions that are successful in taming the tongue.

3. Give an example of how your words have come back to haunt you, perhaps from a social media post. What did you learn from that experience?

4. How do you represent God's kingdom by your words and the pictures you post online?

5. Discuss how we're accountable for our words—both spoken and written.

6. What does your speech say about you? What does your children's speech say about you?

7. Discuss the role of social media in the church.

8. What does metastatic mean in regards to gossip?

9. What kind of ambassador are you?

10. Discuss the meaning of "ill-gotten gain" and Proverbs 20:17.

11. Discuss Proverbs 18:8. What does *inmost body* mean?

10

Pass the Salt

You are the salt of the earth; but if the salt loses its flavor, how shall it be seasoned? It is then good for nothing but to be thrown out and trampled underfoot by men (Matthew 5:13).

Like carbs, salt has a bad reputation because of its excessive use. "On average, American adults eat more than 3,400 milligrams of sodium daily—more than double the American Heart Association's recommended limit of 1,500 milligrams. . . . Excess sodium increases a person's risk for high blood pressure, which can lead to heart disease and stroke."[37] Remember the example of the Applebee's appetizer in Chapter 2? Although the daily guidelines dictate 1,500 to 2,400 milligrams, this one item was 5,480 milligrams. But salt has a lot of good qualities too.

- Historically salt was traded for gold.

- Salt adds flavor to bland foods.
- Salt is used to clean wounds.
- Salt is gargled to clear phlegm.
- Salt is used to clear ice and snow from roads.
- Before refrigeration, salt was used heavily in canning to preserve foods.
- The positively charged particle—the salt ion, Na+(Sodium)—is necessary for life.[38] If it gets watered down or washed out, there can be life-threatening consequences.
- Salt acts and operates deep inside our bodies at the cellular level through osmosis. It literally causes our very hearts to beat.
- Abijah reminded Jeroboam and all of Israel of a salt-covenant given to David (2 Chronicles 13:5).

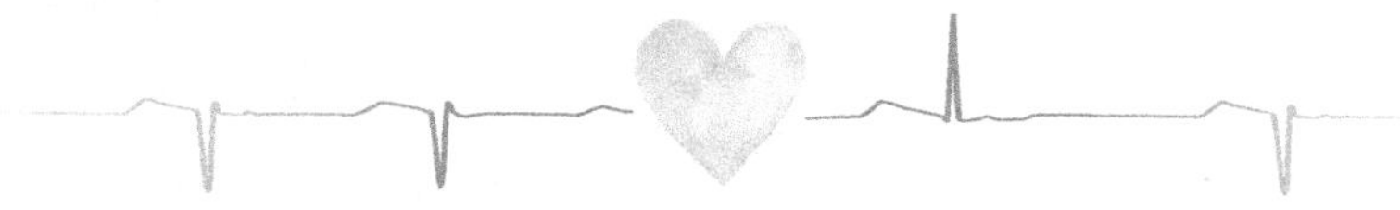

"Should you not know that the Lord God of Israel gave the dominion over Israel to David forever, to him and his sons, by a covenant of salt?" (2 Chronicles 13:5).

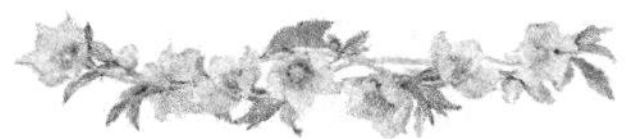

A Little Salt Goes a Long Way

You never know how far-reaching the little things you do or say make someone feel, especially when that person is hurting.

When our son was two, we were expecting our second child with all the hope and joy and planning that goes along with pregnancy. I was not prepared for the obstetrician to tell me that our little baby was

dead. How could that be? How could I look pregnant and feel fine when my baby was dead? The news was devastating, but the wait to miscarry was intolerable. After two weeks, the doctor said I would need to go into the hospital and have the dead baby manually removed. It was almost a relief that I no longer would have to walk around in that state.

Lying on that cold gurney, gowned and prepped for surgery, I felt alone. I don't remember how the nurse looked as she rolled me to the operating room or what her name was, but I do remember her gentle pat on my head.

Like that nurse's gentle pat, non-verbal communications often say more than words. Just being there with those who are hurting and being an active listener is often the most remembered and helpful thing you can do. Don't underestimate the power of a comforting hug or gesture. I am sure the nurse in that small hospital in Raleigh has no memory of me or of the comfort she gave me on that mournful day. It would likely surprise her to know that she made an impression on me at all.

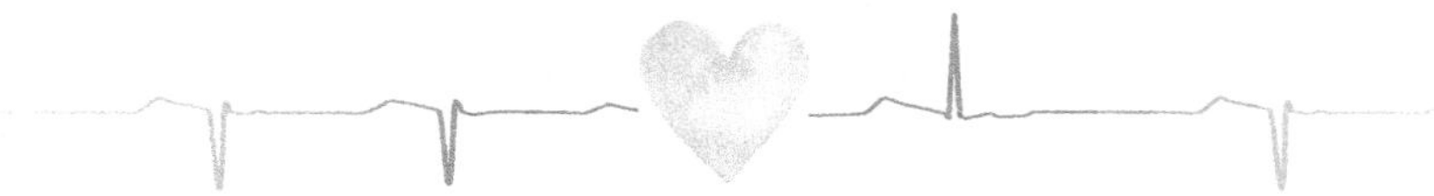

"A little leaven leavens the whole lump"
(Galatians 5:9).

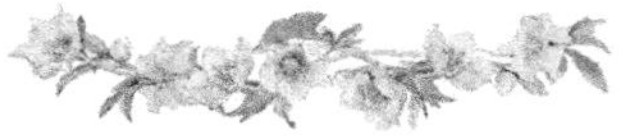

The "Salty" Touch

I am convinced today, with all the modern conveniences of phones and online services, that we could stay in our homes indefinitely. We can order groceries, bank, shop, pay bills, send emails, and fill prescriptions and have them delivered and never have any human contact. Modern technology can be isolating and unhealthy.

In the 1940s, when Hitler was beginning to sweep across Europe, Austrian psychoanalyst René Spitz is believed to have been the first to study institutionalized orphans in Western Europe. From the 1920s the death rate was known to have been extremely high in an orphanage, but that was blamed on contagious diseases. Sterile sheets were placed between the cribs to isolate the children from each other.

To test his theory, Spitz compared the babies in the orphanage to infants raised in isolated hospital cribs in a prison by their own incarcerated mothers. What he found is that 37 percent of the institutionalized babies in the orphanage died, but none of the prison babies did.

The prison babies were better in every way. The orphan infants were found to be scrawny, cognitively, developmentally, psychologically, and behaviorally behind. Why? Spitz theorized that parental love and touch and interaction with the prison moms made the difference. The orphans had only their physical needs met. Their emotional/spiritual needs were not met. Remember, Spitz studied the orphan and prison babies before strict research study guidelines were in place to protect them. This study would never have occurred today. He theorized that the lack of love and parental contact was killing the infants. Sweeping changes in institutional care and ethics and in research studies resulted.[39] John Bowlby and others followed up with further studies.

Babies aren't the only ones who need human relationships and touch. Adults do too. Little kindnesses add flavor to life, and you can't have too much of that. A kind word, a good deed, each thoughtful act is like a grain of salt—it makes life more palatable for someone else.

There is a tendency to ignore the elderly. Many heart patients feel alone, even when they have children in the area. When I ask where their children are, they usually reply, "They are so busy with their own lives." The lyrics of Harry Chapin's 1974 song, "Cat's in the Cradle," come to mind. Too many of us spend our most productive years on the job and then sit down in our easy chairs to find that the children have

grown up and moved away. Children grow up very quickly, although it does not seem so when parents are struggling with the day-to-day responsibility of caring for them. Without your saying a word, children learn what is important to you by your example.

Be mindful of your parents and grandparents and other elderly acquaintances who are alone. They no doubt worked hard to provide for those they loved. As they age, most of their closest friends and family move away or die. The hug you give a widow or widower at church this week may be the only hug they get until the next time they see you. You never know what a difference that kind of asexual touch, kindness, and influence can have on the quality of their lives and yours.

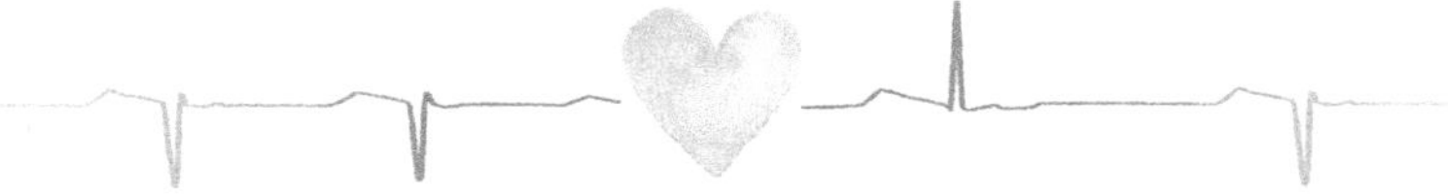

"Then they also brought infants to Him that He might touch them; but when the disciples saw it, they rebuked them. But Jesus called them to Him and said, 'Let the little children come to Me, and do not forbid them; for of such is the kingdom of God' " (Luke 18:15–16).

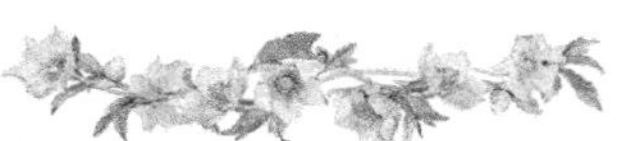

What Are You Dishing Out?

People watch Christians not only to see what we put into our mouths and minds but also to see how we treat others, especially in times of trouble. Too often the person living near to us has never known a member of the Lord's church. We are ambassadors for the Lord's church. Do we act like we are from the kingdom of God? Would there be enough evidence to convict you in a court of law of being a Christian?

What are we reflecting to God and others in our speech, appearance, and attitudes? Solomon says, "As in water face reflects face, so a man's heart reveals the man" (Proverbs 27:19). How can we influence and lead others to Christ if we are perceived unfriendly, cliquish, clannish, impersonal, uncaring, hostile, or indifferent? Only 10 percent of what we communicate are the actual words that we say. The other 90 percent of our message consists of mannerisms and other nonverbal actions. Good communication involves being a good, active listener. How many times have we assumed things and jumped to the wrong conclusions? Learning to be a good listener, to ask open-ended questions, and to read between the lines are skills that can help us understand and lead others to our Lord.

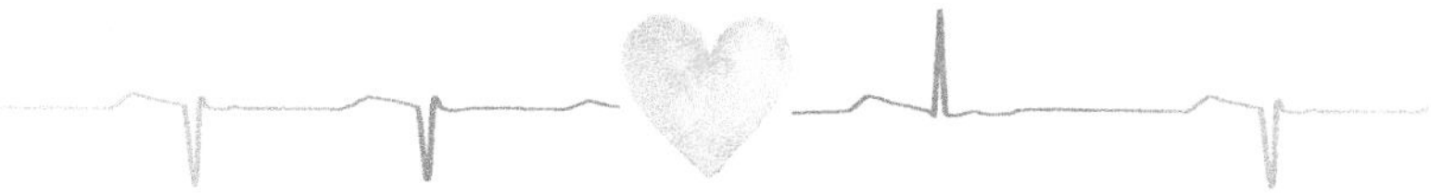

"Can flavorless food be eaten without salt? Or is there *any* taste in the white of an egg?" (Job 6:6).

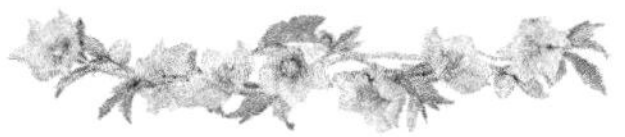

A Scowl or a Smile

What we say may be perceived very different from what we intend while on the job, out in the world, in interactions with our sisters, or with any authority figures. Our hearts will tell on us. Are we reflecting godly attitudes daily? Poor communication of the love of God can cause us to lose our influence on others and actually drive people away from the church.

Remember, people often "mirror back" your own smile or scowl. A genuine smile is inviting and reflects warmth and welcome. It is the small things in life that often leave an impression.

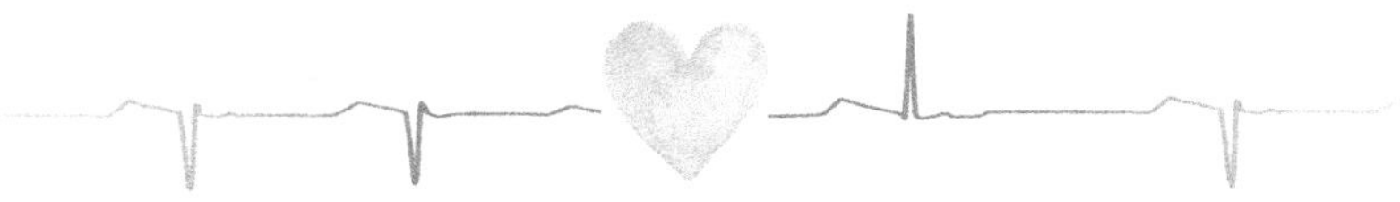

"Let your speech always be with grace, seasoned with salt, that you may know how you ought to answer each one" (Colossians 4:6).

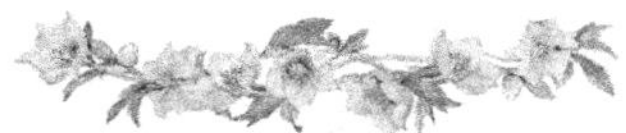

Let's be careful what we dish out and how we dish it out. We do not know how far our influence will reach. When we lose our patience in the grocery store or on the job or show an unloving, impatient attitude toward those we meet, how can we influence them to the Lord?

"Well-chosen kind words are just like salt. They can actually melt hearts."[40] Our speech must be controlled from deep inside our hearts. We must be aware of the far-reaching effects of what we say and do. We do influence those around us whether we want to or not.

Are You a Carrot, an Egg, or a Coffee Bean?[41]

A young woman came to her grandmother and said. "I can't take it anymore. My life is a mess. It is too hard dealing with my husband, children, and a job."

Without saying a word, the grandmother turned on the stove and put on three pots of water. As the pots began to boil, she put a carrot into the first pot, an egg into the second one, and some ground coffee beans into the third one.

After twenty minutes, she took them off the stove and asked her granddaughter to touch the softened carrot, peel the egg

and feel the once-liquid inside now hardened. Then she asked her to sip the coffee.

The granddaughter smiled as she inhaled the rich aroma and tasted the deep flavor of the coffee. The granddaughter said, "I see carrots, an egg, and some coffee. What is this about, Grandma?"

The grandmother explained. Each of these three objects faced the same adversity—boiling water. Each reacted differently.

The carrot went in strong, hard, and unrelenting. After being subjected to the boiling water, it became soft and weak. The liquid part of the egg, protected by a fragile shell, had become hardened in the boiling water. The ground coffee beans were unique, however. They changed the water. The grandmother asked her granddaughter, "Which are you?"

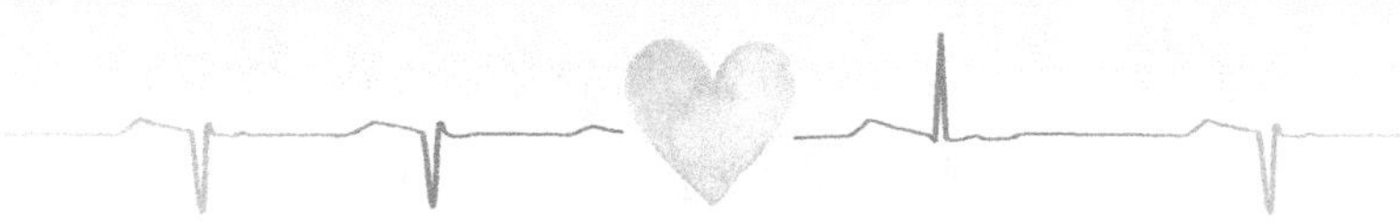

"You are the salt of the earth; but if the salt loses its flavor, how shall it be seasoned? It is then good for nothing but to be thrown out and trampled underfoot by men" (Matthew 5:13).

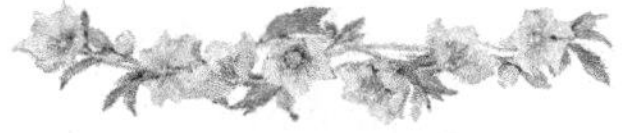

When adversity comes knocking at your door, how do you respond? Are you a carrot, an egg, or a coffee bean? When pain and adversity come, do you wilt and lose your strength? Are you like the egg? The shell looks the same, but after a death, financial hardship, or

some other trial, do you become hardhearted and stiff? Or are you like the coffee beans that changed the water? The very circumstance that brought the adversity, pain, and hardship to that third pot changed its contents into something quite wonderful. The hot water caused the coffee to release its fragrance and flavor. If you are like the coffee, when things are at their worst, you can be the force that changes someone else's life, and you can do that through even the smallest of deeds—like a tiny grain of salt. So are you like an egg, a carrot, or a coffee bean?

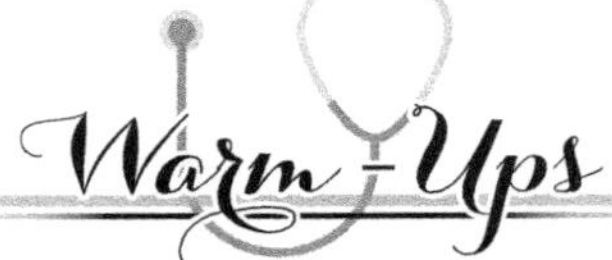

Warm-Ups

Fill a glass bowl with water. Drop a pebble into the center and watch the wave action. Discuss how this demonstrates our influence and words.

Soul Stretches

Spread a few grains of salt this week. Choose two people you can share a scripture with, two people to hug, and send two notes of encouragement to someone in your church bulletin who is struggling. Share the results with the class.

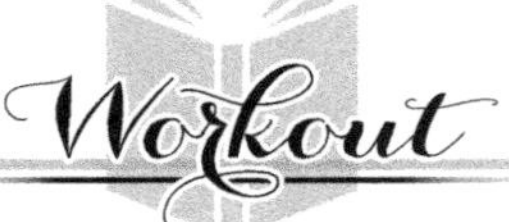

Workout

1. What does the Bible say about salt (Matthew 5:13)?

2. List some verbal and nonverbal ways we influence others?

3. Discuss the role of an ambassador. What would an ambassador of the Lord's church look like?

4. Research and discuss the symptoms of a low-sodium diet.

5. Thinking about salt as a "sodium pump," how can we be salty in the church?

11

Desire True Milk

These [the Bereans] were more fair-minded than those in Thessalonica, in that they received the word with all readiness, and searched the Scriptures daily to find out whether these things were so (Acts 17:11).

Remember the advertising campaign, "Got Milk?" The hope was that the ads, using celebrities and athletes wearing milk moustaches, would encourage people to drink milk. The ads touted the benefits of milk: calcium to strengthen bones and protein to build muscles.

Growth Demands Change

Dairy is a basic food group that is good for our bones and teeth. Dairy products, such as milk, cheese, and yogurt, are linked to lower the risk of heart disease and type 2 diabetes, as well as lower blood pressure.

The important nutrients in dairy include vitamin D, calcium, potassium, and protein.[42] In a groundbreaking 2016 article in *Circulation*, some evidence now suggests that dairy fat may not be as dangerous to the heart as we first thought.[43] It suggests that whole milk may actually be better for type 2 diabetics due to gastric emptying and biochemical reactions. More information will surely follow.

A mother's milk is perfectly suited to meet all her newborn's nutritional needs. Babies breastfeed for a relatively short time, because breast milk will not meet the nutritional requirements of a growing toddler. Changing a child's diet to solid food is essential for growth and development. Our nursing babies soon want to eat from the table.

It is just as important that babes in Christ turn from milk to solid food in their growth as Christians. We must be willing to change and grow.

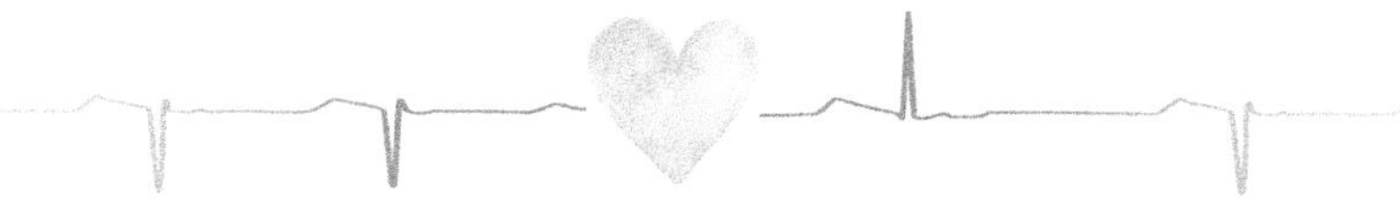

"For though by this time you ought to be teachers, you need someone to teach you again the first principles of the oracles of God; and you have come to need milk and not solid food" (Hebrews 5:12).

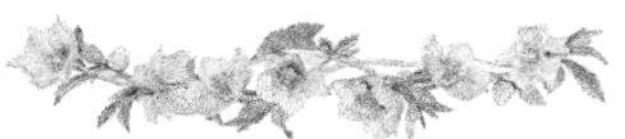

The Constant Is Change

During orientation on my first job as a new, very green nurse, one of my instructors asked me how I was doing. I said, "Great! Everything is perfect." He said, "You are in the honeymoon phase of employment. I want you to remember one thing, 'The only thing you can count on in health care is change.'" I have come to believe that statement is true,

not only about health care but also life in general. And change can be painful.

In sixth grade, my leg bones ached. Later I noticed I was taller than almost anyone in my class. I had been experiencing growing pains! Although painful, change can promote much-needed growth.

In order to grow spiritually, we must not become complacent. We need to be challenging our minds constantly toward transformation.

> And do not be conformed to this world, but be transformed by the renewing of your mind, that you may prove what is that good and acceptable and perfect will of God (Romans 12:2).

Change is inevitable. Although we like to be comfortable and normally hate changes, we must be willing, like the caterpillar, to come out of our cocoon and become a butterfly in order to fly.

Think of the change in technology over the years. We can now reach people in remote places that we could never reach before. Is learning how to use this technology an easy process? For most of us the answer is no. The process is a painful one. Change can be painful but it can be a spark for growth.

What kind of spark does it take to get me from a lukewarm Christian to a red-hot Christian? Is change what is needed? Am I renewing my mind?

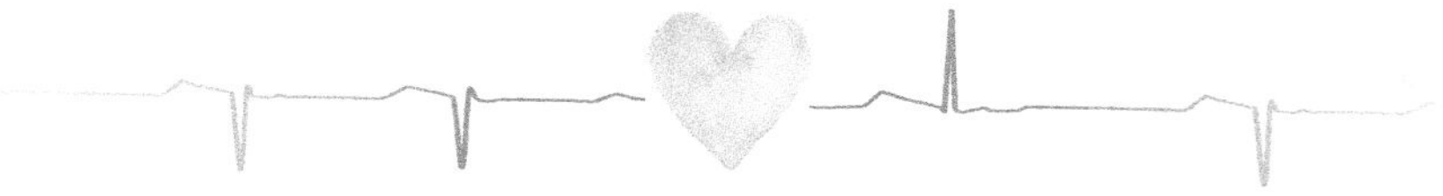

"Therefore, laying aside all malice, all deceit, hypocrisy, envy, and all evil speaking, as newborn babes, desire the pure milk of the word that you may grow thereby, if indeed you have tasted that the Lord is gracious" (1 Peter 2:1–3).

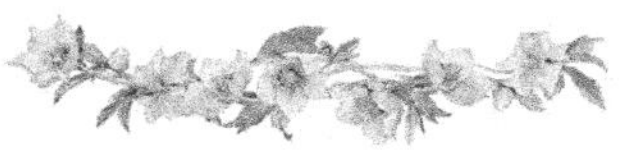

Growth Formula:
Desire, Discipline, and Digging

Desire

The word *desire,* per *Strong's Dictionary,* means to crave intensely or to long for. This earnest craving must come from your heart. In Matthew 5:6, Jesus says "Blessed are those who hunger and thirst for righteousness, for they shall be filled."

Today you can buy many varieties of milk that meet your nutritional needs—whole, two percent fortified, one percent, skim, and others. When Peter says to desire the "pure milk of the word," he is letting us know there is only one milk that will meet our spiritual needs. And this milk, the Word, will strengthen us because we know God "is able to do exceedingly abundantly above all that we ask or think" (Ephesians 3:20).

Discipline

Paul must have observed the athletic runners, possibly in Greece, train and discipline their bodies to compete and win a race. The coveted prize back then was an olive branch. He encourages us to run our race of life to win an imperishable prize in heaven.

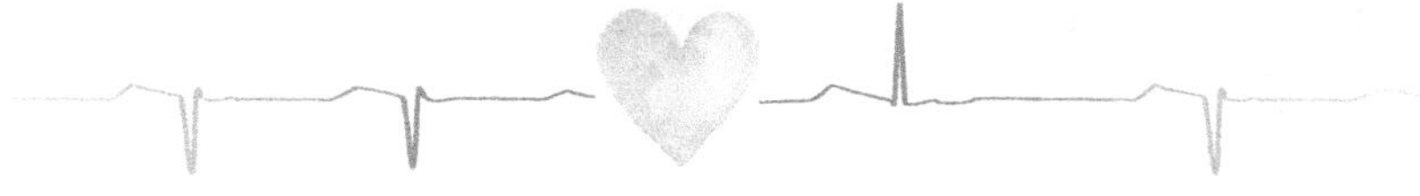

"Run in such a way that you may obtain it. And everyone who competes for the prize is temperate in all things. Now they do it to obtain a perishable crown, but we for an imperishable crown. Therefore, I run thus: not with uncertainty. Thus, I fight: not as one who beats the air. But I discipline my body and bring it into subjection, lest, when I have preached to others, I myself should become disqualified" (1 Corinthians 9:24–27).

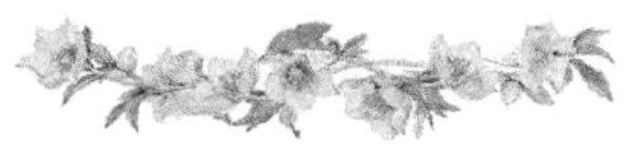

Most Christians have the proper nourishment from the Word, readily available—an open Bible, iPad, study tools, and commentaries. But these tools do not transmit by wireless impulses into the brain. Paul's admonition is to *run*. Only a disciplined runner wins the prize.

Digging in the Word

Infants won't grow if they are never nourished by anything but breast milk or formula. At first, infants may spit and choke on a bite of solid food but with practice they soon master the technique of swallowing cereal and soft strained foods. Then with additional practice, they soon master a fork and spoon to eat more solid food. In order to grow spiritually we must "grow in grace and knowledge of our Lord" (2 Peter 3:18). The only way to do that is to study and rightly divide the word of truth (2 Timothy 2:15). Verse 23 warns us, however, to avoid foolish and ignorant disputes, and the subsequent strife that follows.

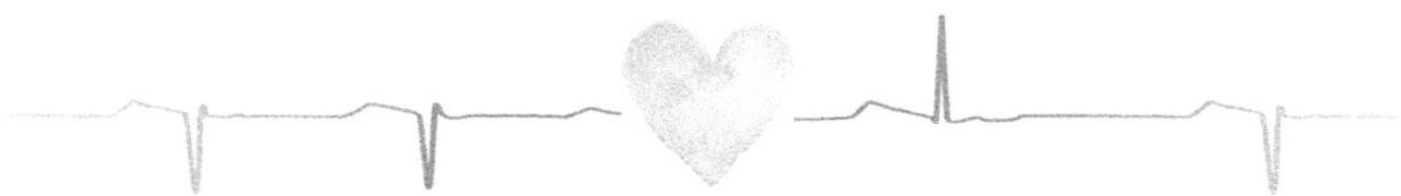

"For everyone who partakes only of milk is unskilled in the word of righteousness, for he is a babe. But solid food belongs to those who are of full age, that is, those who by reason of use have their senses exercised to discern both good and evil" (Hebrews 5:13–14).

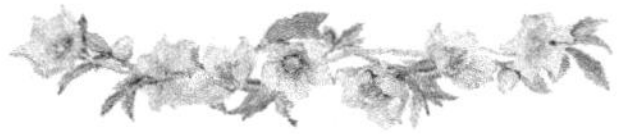

Don't Look Back

Satan wants us to get bogged down with past baggage. Let's throw off the chains of sins that weigh us down and run our life race with endurance (Hebrews 12:1). An endurance race takes discipline. First-time

marathon runners do not usually win or even qualify. It takes time and training and discipline to increase their endurance. Paul also says to forget those things behind us, reach forward to things ahead, and press on toward the goal (Philippians 3:12–14). If you have ever watched the Olympic runner winners, you probably have noticed that they never look back.

Chapter 4 of the book of Philippians is one of the most encouraging chapters in the Bible. Paul encourages,

- Do not be anxious (v. 6).
- Pray to God and the peace of God which surpasses all understanding will guard your hearts and minds through Christ Jesus (vv. 6–7).
- Meditate on true, noble, just, pure, lovely, reputable, virtuous, and praiseworthy things (v. 8).

In Philippians 4:13 he says, "I can do all things through Christ who strengthens me" and ends the chapter with, "And my God shall supply all your need according to His riches in glory by Christ Jesus" (v. 19).

Measure Your Soul

To grow spiritually, we must decide to set parameters, make time for God, and reflect about ourselves.

1. *Set Parameters*
   Our bodies are to be used for the Lord. In order to do that, certain guidelines need to be established about what we are consuming.

   —Decide what ideas you will chew on and ingest daily.

   —Pay more attention to the words of the songs you listen to.

—Pay attention to the types of TV programs and movies you are watching.

—Pay attention to the types of books you are reading. Some women's books in the romance genre can be considered soft porn.

—Decide what you are going to feed your family.

—Monitor what your children are doing on home computers.

—Limit the amount of time your children spend each day playing video games and watching TV.

—Eat together at the dinner table, and feed your family wholesome conversation, as well as nutritional meals.

—Take a look at your friends. Remember that "bad company ruins good morals" (1 Corinthians 15:33 ESV). Do your friends encourage you to gossip or engage in social drinking?

2. *Make Time for God*

At work the most common excuse I hear for not exercising and getting heart healthy is this, "I just don't have time." But we always make time for things that are important to us. Our calendars do not lie. Jesus says, "For where your treasure is there your heart is also" (Matthew 6:21). So we must learn to make time for things that are important to God. Asking yourself a few questions can be eye-opening.

—How am I spending my time?

—Am I making God the center of my life?

—How much time am I really spending on spiritual things?

—Am I spending too much time on my appearance, on myself in general, or at work concentrating on a secular job?

—Where am I spending my time? What events block hours and days on my calendar? You may be surprised how little time you actually spend ingesting God's Word.

—Are you just being a pew warmer?

—Are you more interested in the well-being of the community than in the growth of the church?

—Do you take a job to be closer to church activities?

—When you are planning to move, do you shop for a house near a strong church family?

—Is the growth of the church your priority?

—What do others see when they are looking at you? Do they see God in you?

3. *Reflect about Self*
To become spiritual requires self-reflection. The ladies of the Cary Church of Christ recently hosted a ladies' day to examine this issue based on a passage in the book of Malachi that many of us have overlooked over the years.

Reflections[44]

Malachi 3:3 says, "He will sit as a refiner and a purifier of silver." Those in our Bible class were puzzled. What could this statement have to do with the character and nature of God? One class member volunteered to research the matter of processing silver and report to the class.

That week, the woman made arrangements to observe a silversmith at work. She did not tell him about the class discussion. So far as he knew, she was a curiosity seeker, just someone who wanted to know more about the process of refining silver. As she watched, the

skilled artisan put a piece of silver in his ladle and began to heat it over the fire. "In refining silver," he explained, "all impurities have to be burned away, so I am holding the ladle over the fire where the flames are hottest."

The woman thought about God holding us in such a hot spot. Then she thought again about the verse that says: "He sits as a refiner and a purifier of silver."

"Is it true," she asked the silversmith, "that you have to sit there in front of the fire the whole time the silver is being refined?"

"Yes," he answered. "Not only do I have to sit here holding the silver, but I have to keep my eyes on it the entire time. If the silver is left a moment too long in the flames, it will be destroyed."

The woman was silent for a moment. Then she asked the question that had to be asked: "How do you know when the silver is fully refined?"

He smiled at her and answered, "Oh, that's easy. When I see my image in it, I know it is ready."

—Author unknown

Do we reflect our Creator? We must look deep inside our hearts to answer that question.

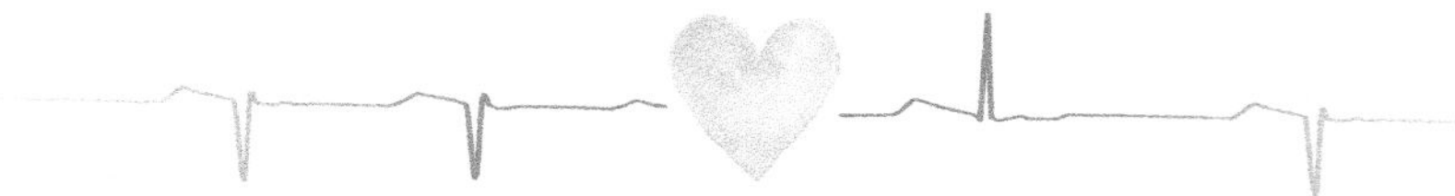

"He will sit as a refiner and a purifier of silver; He will purify the sons of Levi, and purge them as gold and silver, that they may offer to the Lord an offering in righteousness" (Malachi 3:3).

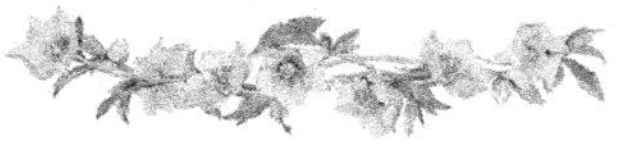

Exercise Tools

Use the Internet positively. Many online study tools and blogs are very helpful for spiritual growth. Check them out.

1. The *Digging Deeper* series is a study available at thecolleyhouse.org and is a great way to enrich your ladies' programs.
2. Olive Tree online Bibles and software are handy ways to dig deeper when you study, and they are at your fingertips. I have a New King James Version of the Bible with a built-in *Strong's Dictionary* on my phone.
3. A great way to grow spiritually is to become a World Bible School or World English Institute online teacher. You can be a world missionary without leaving your living room. Even the homebound can be a missionary.

The Seal of Approval

Jesus said, "Do not labor for the food that perishes, but for the food which endures to everlasting life, which the Son of Man will give you, because God the Father has set His seal on Him" (John 6:27). We can count on Jesus as the authentic Savior. God has put His seal on Him.

I am reminded of the Hanes underwear commercial. The inspector says, "It won't say Hanes until I say it says Hanes." God is promising us that Jesus is stamped with God's seal of approval. In Ephesians 1:13, Paul says,

> In Him you also trusted, after you heard the word of truth, the gospel of your salvation; in whom also, having believed, you were sealed with the Holy Spirit of promise, who is the guarantee of our inheritance until the redemption of the purchased possession, to the praise of His glory.

So Paul is saying if we have trusted and believed the gospel, we are sealed also, guaranteeing our inheritance. Belief requires action. We must set our priorities and obtain that seal of approval. Put first things first.

Take time to evaluate your spiritual diet. Are you making progress or are you stuck in a rut? If you have been a Christian for several years and are still being nourished only by the milk of the Word, it's time to take action. Increase your study time, your participation in Bible classes, and your attentive ear in worship, and move on to solid food. Focus on a more dedicated prayer life, and dig in and become a teacher of the Word.

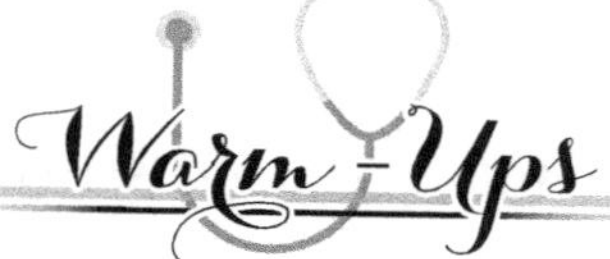

- Share examples of how a negative experience motivated you to change for the better. Then share examples of a positive experience that motivated you to change.
- What other experiences have motivated a change in you? Did the change happen immediately?

Soul Stretches

Look at your calendar. Commit to finding 15 minutes a day you can devote to God in prayer and study. Continue to add 5 minutes to this routine each week until your reach 30 minutes.

1. Has change in your life produced growth? If so, how and why?

2. Is time in the cocoon important to the caterpillar? Why?

3. What other things are necessary to transform our bodies and minds?

4. What does attitude have to do with desire?

5. What does a lukewarm Christian look like and act like?

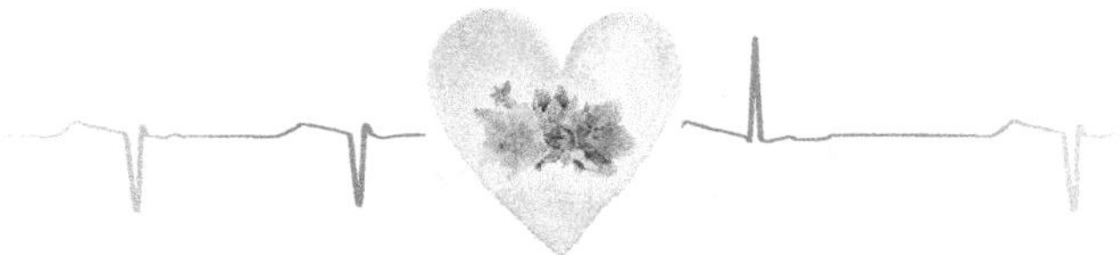

12

Practice Selflessness

Strive to enter through the narrow gate, for many, I say to you, will seek to enter and will not be able (Luke 13:24).

We need to make time for food and nourishment, so we need to fuel up at regular intervals to move about and work efficiently. One of the biggest mistakes my patients make is coming to exercise without eating breakfast. I tell them that is like trying to drive a car with no gas in it. Since they "weigh in," many of them skip breakfast thinking that will reflect in a weight loss.

God's Checks and Balances

Skipping meals tricks your thyroid into thinking you are starving, so it slows down, causing you to put on weight. The thyroid is really good at hanging on to every calorie, if it thinks you are starving. The liver

"dumps" out sugar stores, especially in the middle of the night if it thinks you do not have enough sugar for bodily functions. God has put these checks and balances in place for our own good. We can get into a vicious circle of extreme hunger, overeating, and starving that throws our bodies into a chaotic state. Skipping or skimping on meals does not work and, although often done for weight loss, will have the opposite effect—weight gain.

We must make time for regular spiritual nourishment as well. Are you living a Whack-a-Mole life? Whack-a-Mole is a game you might have played at an arcade. Little mole-like puppets pop up one at a time and your job is to smack them back down with a big mallet. They keep popping up faster and faster. The more moles you whack, the more points you get. Are you beating things down in real life as they pop up but never really getting rid of them or getting ahead?

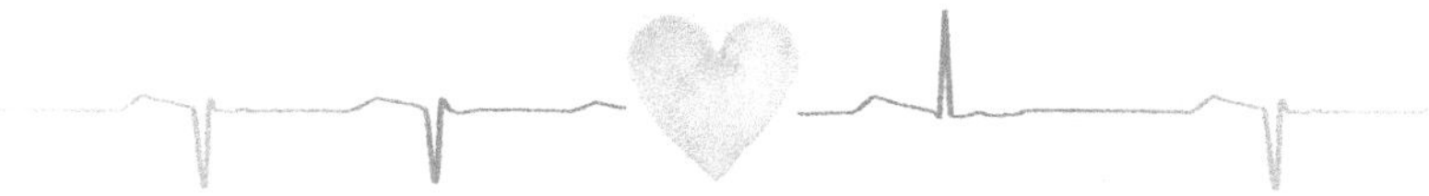

"But when he came to himself, he said, 'How many of my father's hired servants have bread enough and to spare, and I perish with hunger!' " (Luke 15:17).

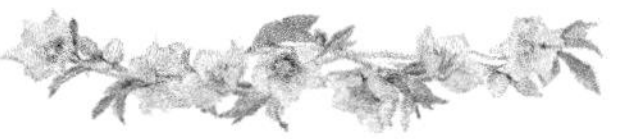

Spiritual Starvation

Are you showing up every now and then to worship, when nothing else important is going on? Skipping worship or skimping on regular Bible study will lead to spiritual starvation. Lack of contact with our brothers and sisters in Christ will grease the wheels of spiritual starvation. When we miss services because of social activities, we teach our

children, without saying a word, that worship is not as important as soccer games, band concerts, or chess matches.

I once heard about an elder who went to visit a man who had neglected worship for several months. This man said, "I can worship God right here from my home." The elder sat down with this man in front of the fireplace where a nice fire was burning. While he and the man talked, the elder took a poker and pulled a single ember out of the fire. As the luster of the ember began to fade, the two men fell silent.

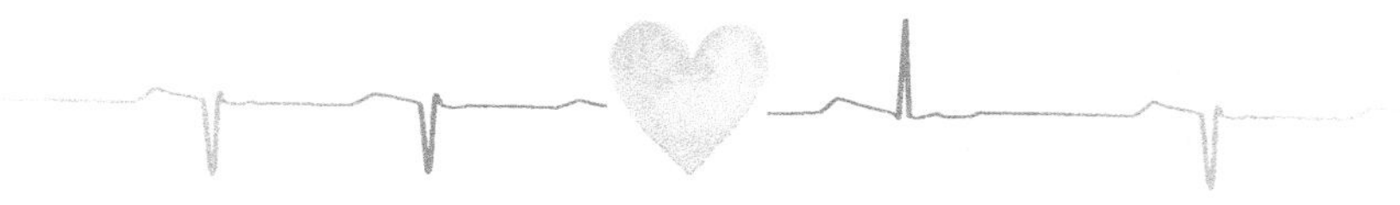

"This being so, I myself always strive to have a conscience without offense toward God and men" (Acts 24:16).

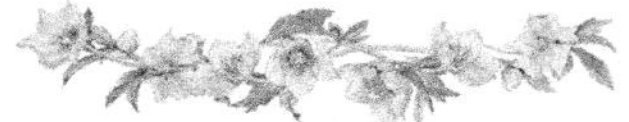

At last the ember lost all its glow. The elder, without saying a word, pushed it back into a nest of glowing embers. Immediately the red glow began to return. Working with the other embers, it helped to make the flame hotter. The weak brother broke the silence: "I'll be there Sunday." Yes, we need each other to keep the flame hot.

Take Smaller Bites

If you do not like how your life is going, you have two choices. You can do nothing and live with things the way they are, or you can grab the bull by the horns and begin to make needed changes. It is all about choices. It is important to look at your life and set realistic goals. Try breaking big goals into smaller pieces. For example, if I told you, "You need to lose 60 pounds to be healthy," that may seem too far out of

reach. But if I said, "Lose one pound a week by cutting out sweet tea and desserts, exercise 30 minutes a day, five days a week, and drink more water," that is much more attainable and reasonable.

Getting physically fit and setting physical goals is important in order to do the work of the Lord daily, but getting spiritually fit and setting spiritual goals is more important. Our eternal health depends upon it. If, for example, you want to incorporate the fruit of the Spirit (Galatians 5:22–23) into your life, don't try to work on all of them at once. Choose one. Make kindness your goal for the week. And then break that goal into smaller pieces. Here are some thoughts that might help you fulfill that goal:

1. On the first day, look up all the verses in the Bible using the word *kindness*.
2. On the second day, pray that God will help you to be successful in becoming kinder.
3. On the third day, call each member on your sick list.
4. On the fourth day, invite someone to go with you to visit one person on your list.
5. On the fifth day, send a card to another person.
6. On the sixth day, invite a guest for dinner.
7. On the seventh day, entertain the guest you invited yesterday.

What seemed to be a very large nebulous goal became attainable when broken down into seven smaller daily pieces. None of these daily activities required a huge time investment. Select a new aspect of the fruit of the Spirit to work on each month. Even if you do monthly activities instead of daily or weekly ones, you will accomplish something. How are you using the Lord's time He has loaned to you?

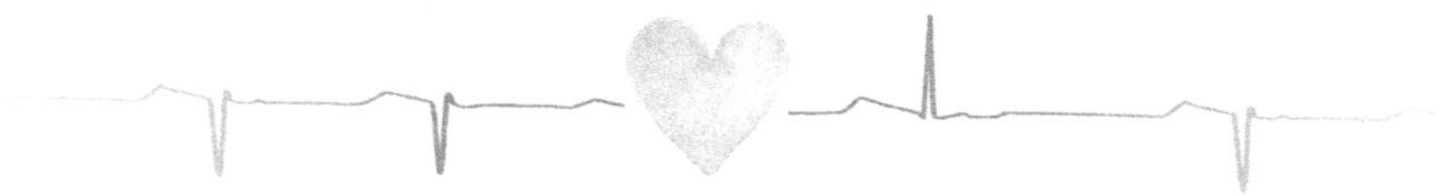

"But those who wait on the Lord shall renew their strength; they shall mount up with wings like eagles, they shall run and not be weary, they shall walk and not faint" (Isaiah 40:31).

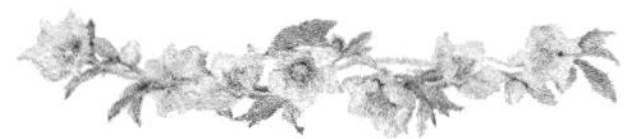

Attitude Matters

Would you agree that the choices we make in food, entertainment, and activities affect and influence those around us, especially our children? Desire and choose some type of real soul food to buff up the body and the soul. The key to optimum physical and spiritual health is 90 percent attitude and 10 percent ability.

Zig Zigler was known for the slogan "attitude determines altitude." Paul's attitude helped him to soar spiritually:

> Not that I speak in regard to need, for I have learned in whatever state I am to be content: I know how to be abased, and I know how to abound. Everywhere and in all things I have learned both to be full and to be hungry, both to abound and to suffer need. I can do all things through Christ who strengthens me (Philippians 4:11–13).

Paul lived with limitations in his life. None of us can do everything perfectly all the time, but we can all do something. "I am only one, but still I am one. I cannot do everything, but still I can do something."[45]

Set a spiritual goal today. How about a goal of becoming more compassionate? Take someone for coffee. Write someone an encouraging text. A good deed doesn't have to cost a fortune.

Sisters, we need each other desperately. There is no reason to be alone. Reach out to someone today. Let's look to our Father in heaven

to give us the comfort and nourishment we need from Him. He is the only true source. Pray for guidance right now.

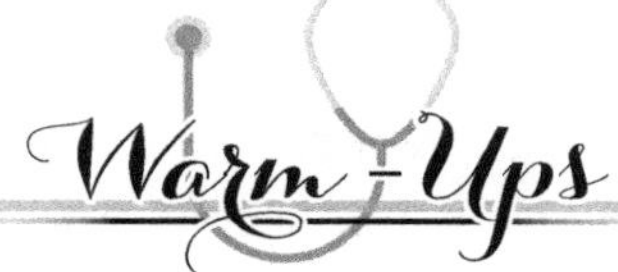

Warm-Ups

Choose a goal today, write out small steps you can take to complete it on your calendar. Share your successes and failures with the class next week.

Soul Stretches

- In light of Philippians 4:11–13, make a contentment list. Evaluate your list. How much is physical and how much is spiritual?
- Challenge yourself with contentment that is in all things and everywhere. Why do we need the strength of Christ for true contentment?

Workout

1. Why is skipping meals, whether physical or spiritual, dangerous and unhealthy?

2. Are you living a whack-a-mole life? If so, what steps can you take to correct it?

3. How can you practically incorporate physical and spiritual exercise into your life? Specifically, what steps can you take?

4. Why does an exercise buddy help?

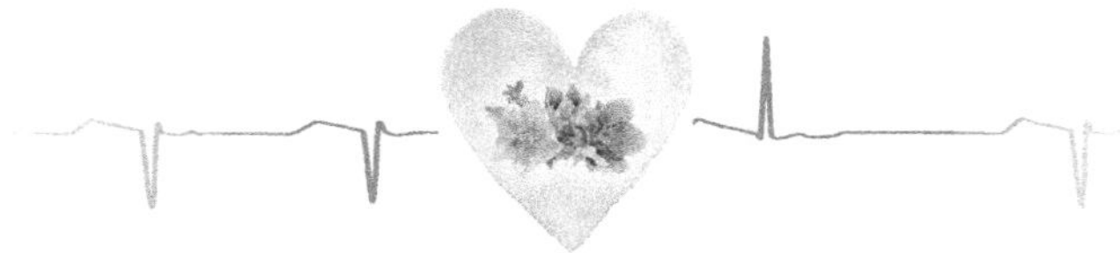

—13—

Hydrate, Hydrate, Hydrate!

This is He who came by water and blood— Jesus Christ; not only by water, but by water and blood. And it is the Spirit who bears witness, because the Spirit is truth (1 John 5:6).

Water for the Heart

You hear about the importance of water almost every day. Hydrate. Hydrate. Hydrate. In the healthy-hearted adult, six to eight glasses (48–64 ounces) a day is generally recommended.[46] Water removes impurities from the blood, helps in digestion and circulation, and supplies energy to get things done. You must have enough water in your system to keep your blood pressure high enough for the heart to squeeze blood to every cell. If you are dehydrated, your well is too dry. The heart then needs to work harder to pump the blood. It meets that demand by speeding up. Water is a heart essential.

Too much water, however, is not good for those who have a weak heart. In patients with heart failure or poor pumping ability, too much water can cause fluid to back up in the lungs and literally drown them.

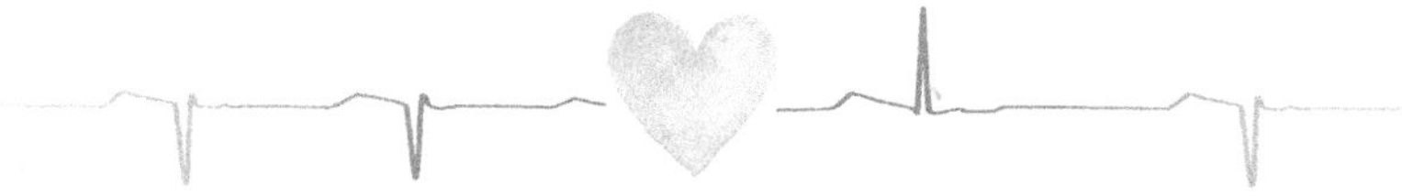

"Once the Divine longsuffering waited in the days of Noah, while the ark was being prepared, in which a few, that is, eight souls, were saved through water" (I Peter 3:20).

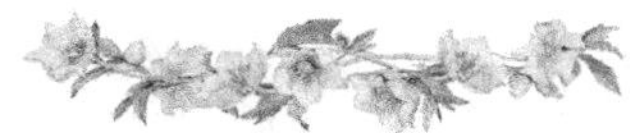

Water for the Soul

After Peter reminds us that in the days of Noah, while the ark was being prepared, eight souls were saved through water, he then explains salvation in Christ in the following verses.

> There is also an antitype which now saves us—baptism (not the removal of filth from the flesh, but the answer of a good conscience toward God), through the resurrection of Jesus Christ, who has gone into heaven and is at the right hand of God, angels and authorities and powers having been made subject to Him (1 Peter 3:21–22).

In the days of Noah, the world was filled with corrupt and unrighteous people who were violent and apparently interested in eating and drinking, marrying and giving in marriage right up until the day Noah entered the ark (cf. Genesis 6:13; Matthew 24:38). All individuals outside the ark were "weak-hearted" in their faith in God. They were drowned. Only the righteous, Noah's family, and the animals in the confines of the ark were saved. By faith, Noah built the ark to God's specifications, not his own. The ark had a door, and that was the only

way to enter. The water carried the ark and all in it to safety. Noah and his family became heirs of righteousness (cf. Hebrews 11:7).

Today the unrighteous are saved by baptism in water, and from that baptism, they are raised from the water as Christ was raised from the grave. They enter the church through that one door and will become heirs of righteousness just as Noah and his family did—by faith. We can learn much from the life of Noah and his obedience.

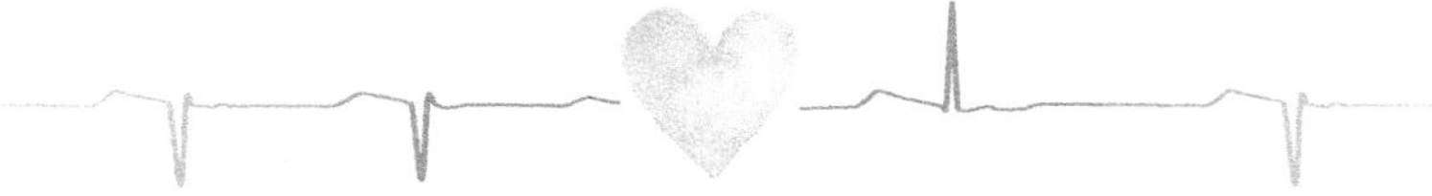

"By faith Noah, being divinely warned of things not yet seen, moved with godly fear, prepared an ark for the saving of his household, by which he condemned the world and became heir of the righteousness which is according to faith" (Hebrews 11:7).

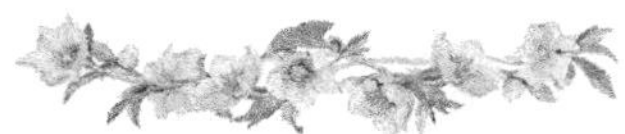

Living Water

We should strive to fill our lives with the *living* water of Jesus Christ. Jesus told the woman at the well that the water He gives is living and would become, in those who receive it, "a fountain of water springing up into everlasting life" (John 4:10–14). The *Strong's Dictionary* definition and meaning of living water is "to have true life and be worthy of the name" or "to be active, blessed, or endless in the kingdom of God" or "having vital power in itself and exerting the same on the soul."

If you have ever done any white-water rafting, you know about the power of a river current. It can be diverted but not easily contained. When water encounters a wall, it searches for tiny crevices through which it begins to seep. As the force of the water creates erosion, the

crevices become larger, finally creating new channels for the water, as it gushes over, under, around, or through the obstacle. Water has the power to carve rivers through mountains!

What powerful imagery Jesus provides! Could our belief in Jesus Christ create an endless current of life? It is no accident that we cannot live without water. God uses our limited understanding of the natural world, along with stories from the Old Testament, to help us comprehend great truths of the New Testament that might otherwise be hidden.

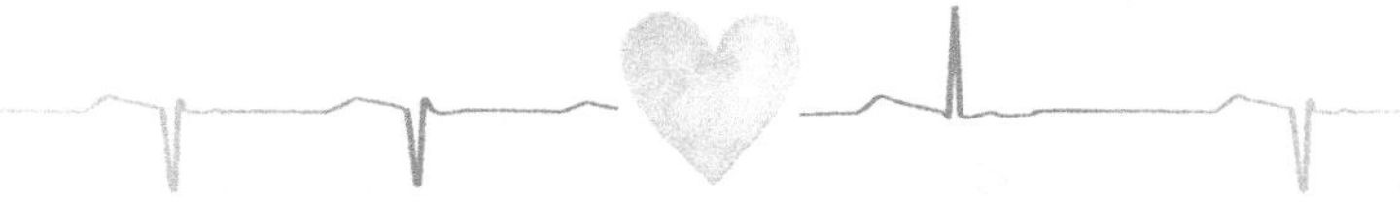

"But the hour is coming, and now is, when the true worshipers will worship the Father in spirit and truth; for the Father is seeking such to worship Him" (John 4:23).

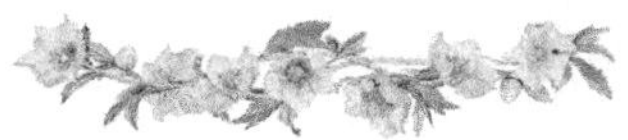

The Power of Blood

Our beating heart and body cannot live without blood. Blood is made up mostly of plasma, which is 92 percent water and solid cells such as red blood cells, white blood cells, and platelets.[47] Blood carries oxygen and nutrition to every cell of our body.[48] Those specialized blood cells respond when we are injured, much like an army responds to a threat. Cells rush to form clots that prevent blood loss. Cells fight infections, carry waste to the liver and kidneys for cleaning, and regulate temperature. Eight to nine percent of our weight is made up of blood. Blood carries hormones. From the hematology society, we also learn blood is a mixture of 55 percent plasma and 45 percent blood cells.

Blood is essential for life. Where does blood come from? "Blood cells develop from hematopoietic stem cells and are formed in the bone marrow."[49] The bone marrow is inside our bones. Interestingly, the bone marrow is mentioned in both the King James Version and the American Standard Version of the Bible. Proverbs 3:7–8 reads, "Be not wise in thine own eyes; fear Jehovah, and depart from evil. It will be health to thy navel and marrow to thy bones" (KJV).

The navel is where the preborn baby's umbilical cord that supplies food and oxygen from its mother is attached. The blood and tissue of the umbilical cord stores stem cells that have the potential of growing into organs. For example, there is a cell in the pancreas that produces insulin. Much research is being done to see if these cells can be transplanted into a person with type 1 diabetes so he can produce insulin again. I am convinced we may live to see a cure for this type of diabetes.

Stem Cells

Perhaps you are familiar with cord blood banks for the storing of infants' umbilical cords.[50] Although stem cells have gotten a negative connotation, we all have stem cells. When we are born, there is a high percentage of them in the umbilical cord that previously has been discarded. Stem cells are genetically related to your baby and family and are "dominant cells in the way they contribute to the development of all tissues, organs, and systems in the body."[51] The field of Regenerative Medicine is based on the new hope and prayer that eventually children may be able to treat diseases or grow replacement cells for themselves or their siblings from their stem cells. I attended a conference in Raleigh, North Carolina, called "Taking Control of Your Diabetes" and learned from the endocrinologists that strides are being made with the pancreatic islet of Langerhans insulin-producing cells.

The hope is these cells can be "grown" and transplanted to potentially end type 1 diabetes as we know it. Perhaps in my lifetime, we can find an end to type 1 diabetes.

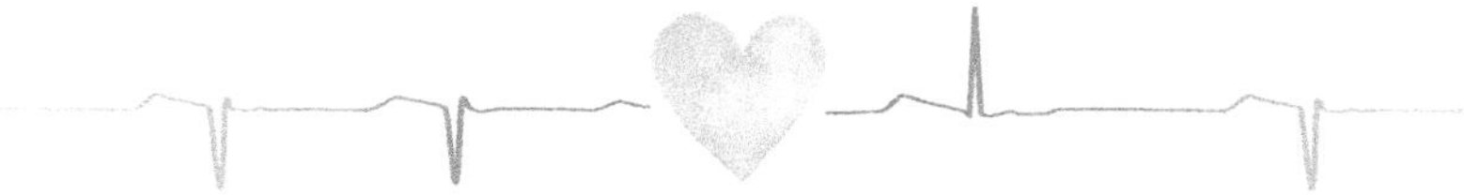

"Trust in the Lord with all thine heart; and lean not unto thine own understanding. In all thy ways acknowledge him, and he shall direct thy paths. Be not wise in thine own eyes: fear the Lord, and depart from evil. It shall be health to thy navel, and marrow to thy bones" (Proverbs 3:5–8 KJV).

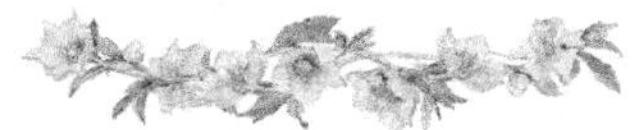

Fearing God Is Healthy

Health in Proverbs 3:8 means "healing," while *navel*, in a figure of speech, means the "center." *Marrow* means "refreshment" or a "drink." We now know that bone marrow makes red blood cells that are replaced every 120 days. Solomon was born about a thousand years before Christ. Rudimentary microscopes were not invented until the late sixteenth century, a little more than 400 years ago. So how could Solomon have known that the bone marrow is responsible for making the very cells that compose the blood or that they were replaced periodically by bone marrow?

Only in relatively recent times has the medical field even been aware of the role bone marrow plays in making blood cells and its relationship to stem cells. Solomon's knowledge had to come from God, the creator of all things. The blood cells are made inside the bones in the bone marrow. Blood is essential for life. It is core and fundamental

to life physically and spiritually. We often hear how important it is to exercise the core. You cannot get more core than this!

Sisters, it is no accident our physical bodies cannot live without water or blood. Through water and blood, our cells receive the oxygenated blood and nutrition essential for survival. The only way we can survive eternally is by submission to Him who made the ultimate sacrifice on the cross. We access the benefits of our Lord's sacrifice through faith when we are immersed in water (baptized) for the remission of sins (Mark 16:16; Romans 6:3; Colossian 2:11–12). The blood of Jesus purchased the church (Acts 20:28). Blood is core to eternal life.

The Final Challenge

Are you now challenged to do a little contemplation about your life? Are you motivated to develop a diet filled with real soul food, a goal-centered action, and an exercise plan to facilitate your physical and spiritual health? I pray that you are. Solomon reveals the recipe for life and the prescription from God for "health to your flesh and strength to your bones."

I pray to God that you will take what you have learned here and shape up both physically and spiritually. We need more strong, balanced, and stable Christians. A patient wore a T-shirt that said,

Eat right.
Exercise.
Die anyway.

How true. But how we live and how we die are important because of the influence we have on others. Nothing is more important than leading others to Christ. It is like giving sight to a blind person, leading one from darkness to light. The truth is, we have a Great Physician to guide us, and He has already given us His inspired—God-breathed—Word

and direction. Choose God's Word to savor. It contains the real soul food ingredients and the recipe and prescription for life now and life eternally. Medicine left on the shelf or at the pharmacy does your body no good. Take your medicine as prescribed by the Great Physician.

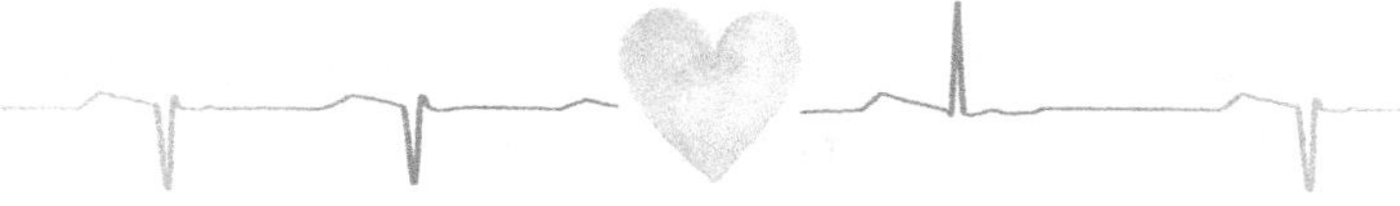

"Trust in the Lord with all of your heart, and lean not on your own understanding" (Proverbs 3:5).

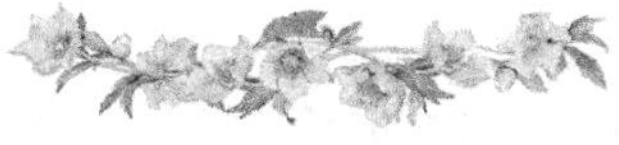

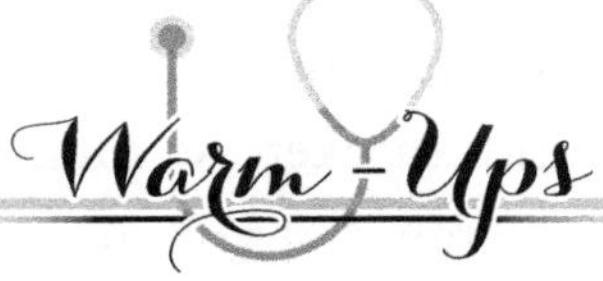

Warm-Ups

- Research the role that water and blood play in your body in relationship to blood pressure and heart rate. What makes up blood?
- Research the Churches of Christ Disaster Relief effort, www.disasterreliefeffort.org. Find out if there is a need for water. Ask your elders if you may help in this area.
- Contact the Red Cross and host a blood drive at your congregation.

Soul Stretches

When was the last time you visited the baptistry at your church building? Ask the elders if it is okay for your ladies' class to visit the area. Try to imagine how someone who is new to the church and about to take on

Christ feels as he or she is about to enter the waters of baptism. What can you do to make the experience better? Take a look around you. Are the changing rooms clean and fresh? What kind of condition are the baptismal garments in? If you, as a class, find there are some improvements you can help make, check with your elders and then do them.

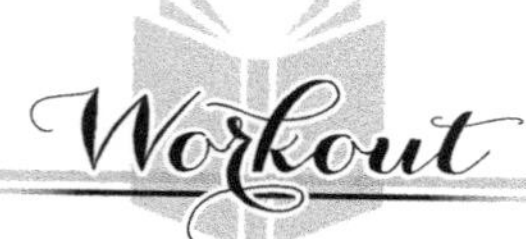

Workout

1. Jesus spoke in parables about sowers and birds and bread, all of which were commonly understood. Why did He do this?

2. In what ways is Jesus the Great Physician? What qualities does He possess?

3. What kind of medicine does Jesus prescribe spiritually?

4. How could Solomon know anything about bone marrow and blood?

5. Highlight or underline each verb (action word) in Proverbs 3:5–8. Look up the meaning of each of these words and discuss. In verse 5 does the word *trust* imply blind trust?

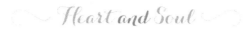

6. What is important about water and blood physically and spiritually?

---

7. What is the three-part advice from Solomon in Proverbs 3:7?

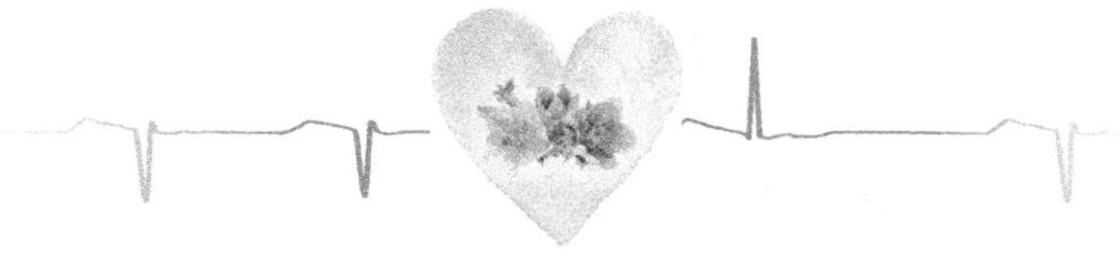

Endnotes

1. A. C. Allen, "Countries Spending the Most on Health Care," *USA Today* (July 7, 2014), accessed November 9, 2014, http://www.usatoday.com/story/money/business/2014/07/07/countries-spending-most-health-care/12282577.
2. "Life Expectancy in the US Rising Slower Than Elsewhere, Says OECD," The Organization for Economic Cooperation and Development (2013), accessed January 6, 2015, http://www.oecd.org/unitedstates/Health-at-a-Glance-2013-Press-Release-USA.pdf.
3. "Heart Disease and Stroke," Healthy People 2020 (October 30, 2014), accessed October 30, 2014, http://www.healthypeople.gov/2020/topics-objectives/topic/heart-disease-and-stroke.
4. "Diet and Lifestyle Recommendations," American Heart Association (September 15, 2014), accessed October 29, 2014, www.heart.org/HEARTORG/GettingHealthy.
5. "Diet and Lifestyle."
6. "Diet and Lifestyle."
7. "Heart Disease and Stroke."
8. "Diet and Lifestyle."
9. "Diet and Lifestyle."
10. If you have more than 50 pounds to lose, you may need to seek a bariatric doctor to assist you in weight loss.
11. "What Is the DASH Eating Plan?" National Institute of Health (June 6, 2014), accessed November 6, 2014, http://www.nhlbi.nih.gov/health/health-topics/topics/dash.
12. "American Heart Association Backs Current BP Treatments," American Heart Association, Inc. (August 4, 2014), accessed November 1, 2014, http://www.heart.org/HEARTORG/Conditions/HighBloodPressure/PreventionTreatmentofHighBloodPressure/American-Heart-Association-backs-current-BP-treatments_UCM_459129_Article.jsp.
13. "Fats and Cholesterol," Heart Foundation (November 14, 2014), accessed November 14, 2014, https://www.heartfoundation.org.au/healthy-eating/food-and-nutrition/fats-and-cholesterol.
14. "What Is Cholesterol?" National Institute of Health (September 19, 2012), accessed January 21, 2015, https://www.nhlbi.nih.gov/health-topics/high-blood-cholesterol.

15. The information provided for McDonald's and Applebee's is from "Restaurant Nutrition," a free software application that can be easily downloaded to your phone. Many common restaurants are listed with nutritional information for appetizers, entrees, desserts, and drinks.
16. "Counting Calories for Weight Loss," Howstuffworks (n.d.), accessed November 9, 2014, http://health.howstuffworks.com/wellness/diet-fitness/weight-loss/counting-calories-for-weight-loss.htm.
17. "Economics" (2012), Distilled Spirits Council of the United States, accessed November 1, 2014, http://www.discus.org/mobile/economics.
18. "Fact Sheets: Alcohol Use and Your Health," Center for Disease Control and Prevention (October 18, 2016), accessed December 26, 2017, https://www.cdc.gov/alcohol/fact-sheets/alcohol-use.htm.
19. "Flavonoids," whfoods.org, http://whfoods.org/genpage.php?tname=nutrient&dbid=119.
20. "Eric Lawson, who portrayed Marlboro man, dies at 72," Associated Press, *Washington Post* (January 27, 2014), accessed January 7, 2015, http://www.washingtonpost.com/national/eric-lawson-who-portrayed-marlboro-man-dies-at-72/2014/01/27/6662d0aa-8772-11e3-916e-e01534b1e132_story.html
21. "Cirrhosis Overview," MayoClinic.org, accessed April 6, 2016, https://www.mayoclinic.org/diseases-conditions/cirrhosis/symptoms-causes/syc-20351487.
22. "Alcoholic Cardiomyopathy," Medscape.com (December 18, 2014), accessed December 26, 2017, https://emedicine.medscape.com/article/152379-overview#a2.
23. "Impaired Driving: Get the Facts," Center for Disease Control (October, 7 2014) accessed November 2, 2014, http://www.cdc.gov/motorvehiclesafety/impaired_driving/impaired-drv_factsheet.html.
24. "Can antioxidants in fruits and vegetables protect you and your heart?" American Heart Association, Inc. (2014), accessed November 1, 2014, http://www.heart.org/HEARTORG/GettingHealthy/NutritionCenter/HealthyEating/Can-antioxidants-in-fruits-and-vegetables-protect-you-and-your-heart_UCM_454424_Article.jsp 2/7/2013.
25. John Walker, "U.S. Tax Code On-Line," accessed December 26, 2017, https://www.fourmilab.ch/uscode/26usc.
26. "Profiling Food Consumption in America," United States Department of Agriculture. (n.d.), accessed November 2014, http://www.usda.gov/factbook/chapter2.pdf.

27. "Exercise: 7 benefits of regular physical activity," Mayo Foundation for Medical Education and Research (1998–2014), accessed November 2, 2014, https://www.mayoclinic.org/healthy-lifestyle/fitness/in-depth/exercise/art-20048389?pg=1.

28. "Core Exercises: Why you should strengthen your core muscles," Mayo Clinic (July 18, 2014), accessed November 4, 2014, https://www.mayoclinic.org/healthy-lifestyle/fitness/in-depth/core-exercises/art-20044751.

29. "Lessons from Geese" Facts 1–5 can be found floating around the Internet, some saying author unknown and others giving Milton Olson as the original author. An original date for this story could not be found.

30. Enhanced Strong's Dictionary. Strong's Bibles & Concordances for the Olive Tree Bible App (2011). Olive Tree Bible Software, Inc. www.olivetree.com.

31. Enhanced Strong's Dictionary.

32. "Chronic stress puts your health at risk," Mayo Clinic (1998–2014), accessed November 9, 2014, http://www.mayoclinic.org/healthy-living/stress-management/in-depth/stress/art-20046037

33. Enhanced Strong's Dictionary.

34. "Binge Eating Disorder Overview and Statistics," National Eating Disorder Association. (n.d.), accessed November 9, 2014, https://www.nationaleatingdisorders.org/binge-eating-disorder.

35. "Health Effects of Cigarette Smoking," Center for Disease Control and Prevention (April, 24 2014), accessed November 8, 2014, https://www.cdc.gov/tobacco/data_statistics/fact_sheets/health_effects/effects_cig_smoking/index.htm.

36. "Loose lips sink ships," *Wikipedia*. https://en.wikipedia.org/wiki/Loose_lips_sink_ships.

37. "9 out of 10 Americans Eat Too Much Sodium Infographic," American Heart Association, accessed Jan. 13, 2018, https://healthyforgood.heart.org/eat-smart/infographics/9-out-of-10-americans-eat-too-much-sodium-infographic.

38. "Link between sodium, calcium and heartbeat illuminated," *Science Daily* (February 13, 2012), accessed December 30, 2017, http://www.sciencedaily.com/releases/2012/02/120213185645.htm.

39. Virginia Hughes, "The Orphanage Problem," *National Geographic* (July 31, 2013). nationalgeographic.com/2013/07/31/the-orphanage-problem. Accessed December 26, 2017.

40. Nancy Eichman, *Seasoning Your Words* (Nashville: Gospel Advocate Company, 1984), p. 16.

41. Adapted from "Grandma Teaches Important Life Lesson Using a Carrot, Eggs, and Coffee," Barbara Diamond, *Little Things*, accessed December 26, 2017, https://www.littlethings.com/grandma-carrot-eggs-coffee.

42. "Nutrients and Health Benefits," USDA ChooseMYPlate.gov (n.d.), accessed November 5, 2014, https://www.choosemyplate.gov/dairy-nutrients-health.

43. Yakoob MY, et al. "Circulating Biomarkers of Dairy Fat and Risk of Incident Diabetes Mellitus Among Men and Women in the United States in Two Large Prospective Cohorts," *Circulation*, 2016, accessed January 1, 2018, https://www.ncbi.nlm.nih.gov/m/pubmed/27006479.

44. Nancy Missler, "Reflections of His Image: How to Walk in the Spirit," *Personal Update News Journal* (January 2009), accessed December 30, 2017, http://www.khouse.org/articles/2009/831.

45. Edward Everett Hale as it appears in the June 11 entry of *A Year of Beautiful Thoughts* compiled by Jeanie A. B. Greenough (New York: Thomas Y. Crowell & Co., 1902), 172.

46. "Water: How much should you drink every day?" MayoClinic.org (September 5, 2014), accessed November 9, 2104, http://www.mayoclinic.org/healthy-living/nutrition-and-healthy-eating/in-depth/water/art-20044256.

47. "Blood Components: Plasma," American Red Cross, accessed January 4, 2018, https://m.redcrossblood.org/learn-about-blood/blood-components/plasma.

48. "Blood Basics," American Society of Hematology (2015), accessed January 5, 2015, http://www.hematology.org/Patients/Basics.

49. "Red Blood Cells," American Society of Hematology (2015), accessed December 6, 2017, http://www.hematology.org/Patients/Basics.

50. "What are umbilcal cord stem cells?" StemCellsAustralia.edu (2014), accessed November 9, 2014, http://www.stemcellsaustralia.edu.au/About-Stem-Cells/FAQ/What-are-umbilical-cord-stem-cells-.aspx.

51. Viacord.com is one such cord blood banking site.